Student Study Guide
to accompany

CONTEMPORARY NUTRITION

Issues and Insights

Third Edition

GORDON M. WARDLAW, PH.D., R.D., L.D.
Division of Medical Dietetics
The Ohio State University

WCB McGraw-Hill

Boston, Massachusetts Burr Ridge, Illinios Dubuque, Iowa
Madison, Wisconsin New York, New York San Francisco, California St. Louis, Missouri

WCB/McGraw-Hill
A Division of The ***McGraw-Hill*** *Companies*

ISBN 0-8151-9272-X

Printed in the United States of America

10 9 8 7 6 5 4 3 2

PREFACE

Mastering Nutrition

I found four important methods for learning course material and making good examination scores when I was a student. I advise you to do all four. This Student Study Guide to accompany Contemporary Nutrition: Issues and Insights is designed to help you with the last three.

1. **Attend every class period.** This is vital because no book or study guide can substitute for a clear explanation of a term or concept by a professor. In addition, although examinations are based on factual material, they also are greatly influenced by the professor's frame of mind. The student needs to both understand important concepts and categorize those concepts in terms of the relative importance the professor puts on them.

2. **Read the textbook.** You should spend at least one hour outside of class for every hour in class reading your textbook. Underline important points. Write in the margins. Use the book to help you understand the concepts developed in class. Follow along in the Study Guide to practice using those concepts. Ideally, read the relevant sections in the textbook and Study Guide before going to class. You will find that a very helpful exercise.

3. **Use flash cards.** A flash card has a word or concept on one side and a corresponding definition or explanation of the concept on the other side. Using flash cards is a powerful method for learning material because you cannot fool yourself into thinking you know the material. Either you know what's on the other side of that flash card -- or you do not. Simply reading your notes or looking at the underlined sections of your book is not enough. In my 18 years of teaching I have seen students increase their grades significantly once they started using flash cards. I used this system throughout my undergraduate and graduate course work. I even convinced many of my friends in graduate school to use this technique.

> I have included a group of flash cards for every chapter in this Study Guide. Providing information in this form is a key part of the approach this Guide takes. However, these are just a start. Make more flash cards for other concepts you think are important. Review your flash cards every day or two. Before an examination review all of them until you know each one. Before the final examination sit in a chair next to a trash can. Run through your flash cards and discard every one you know, and then keep running through the remainder until all are in the trash. In that way you have efficiently reviewed material from the entire course and are ready to excel in the final examination.

4. Take practice examinations. I always found it helpful to take as many previous examinations from a class as I could. These helped me get into the rhythm of taking tests in that subject and challenged me to apply the terms and concepts I had learned. The practice setting allowed time to look up questions I could not answer. I strove eventually to score all answers correctly.

> This Study Guide includes about 25 practice examination questions per chapter. Consider making up more of your own. It is important not to simply memorize an answer but to understand why an answer is correct and why the others are wrong. In that way practice questions will challenge you to apply the concepts you have learned.

Using This Study Guide

This Study Guide has four major sections for each chapter. First, objectives for the chapter are listed to help focus your attention while reading the chapter. Then important word parts are given to help you master the vocabulary. Next you should review the flash cards (see Appendix A) to reinforce the most important chapter concepts. The review and synthesis activities then help reinforce the chapter concepts as you study chapter tables and figures, provide short answers to questions, perform calculations, and analyze aspects of your diet. Finally, examination questions test you over the terms and concepts in the chapter. Because classroom examinations usually cover four to six chapters, the Study Guide will provide you with about 100-150 sample test questions for each examination.

In all, I think that this Study Guide has a system that will help you learn the text material and do well on examinations. This Guide is not a short cut for learning nutrition or a substitute for reading the textbook or attending class. It does, however, provide a logical means by which to study the material and, in turn, excel in the class.

Gordon Wardlaw

CONTENTS

CHAPTER 1
What You Eat and Why

Begin each new Chapter by reading it straight through while striving to master the following points. Then, start your Study Guide activities.

I. Points to consider

Chapter 1 is designed to allow you to:

1. Define the terms carbohydrate, protein, lipid (fat), alcohol, vitamin, mineral, kilocalorie (kcal), and dietary fiber.

2. Outline the ABCD of nutrition assessment: anthropometric, biochemical, clinical, and dietary.

3. List the major characteristics of the American diet and the areas that often need improvement.

4. Describe how various factors affect our food habits: early experiences, ethnic customs, health concerns, advertising, social class, and economics.

5. Outline the basic units used in the metric system and interpret a percentage value.

II. Word parts

Complete the following exercise using words from Chapter 1 for the examples. This will help you master nutrition vocabulary.

Word part	Meaning	Examples
hydr	water	____________
bi(o)	life	____________
anthrop	man	____________
metr	measure	____________
kilo	1000 times	____________
centi	100 times	____________
milli	1/1000	____________

III. Flash cards

Cut out and review the flash cards for this chapter in Appendix A. These will help you focus on the major points of each chapter.

IV. Review and synthesis

These exercises provide an opportunity for you to practice using knowledge gained from lectures, the textbook, and the flash cards. Check your answers to the questions using the page references for your textbook (in parentheses). Some answers also will be listed near the end of the chapter in this Study Guide. This will be pointed out to you when that is the case.

A. "You have probably heard the terms carbohydrates, protein, lipids (fats and oils), vitamins, minerals. These, plus water, make up the six classes of nutrients found in food." From memory, list some of the essential nutrients in the human diet and their approximate contribution to body weight under the correct category. (5-6)

	ENERGY NUTRIENTS					
	Carbohydrate	Fat	Protein (amino acids)	Vitamins	Minerals	Water
Percentage of body weight						

Refer to Table 1-2 in your text to check your answers, and then use the chapter to add any missing information. Review this exercise again during the next few weeks to refresh your memory. Check your answers and then add any missing information.

B. 1. "Energy is held in the chemical bonds of carbohydrates, fats, proteins, and alcohol." Briefly characterize the energy sources in a diet. Then complete the rest of the table. (6-9,18)

Energy source	Kcal per gram	Percentage of kcal in U.S. diet
Carbohydrate		
Protein		
Fat		
Alcohol		too variable between individuals

2. A piña colada drink may have 15 grams of alcohol, 6 grams of carbohydrate, 1 gram of fat, and 1 gram of protein. How many kcal would it contain? (8)

3. "You can determine what portion of total energy intake is contributed by the various energy-yielding nutrients." Assume that one day you consume 150 grams of carbohydrate, 80 grams of fat, and 60 grams of protein. This consumption yields a total of ______ kcal. The percentage of your total energy intake derived from each nutrient would be: (19)

carbohydrate __________

fat __________

protein __________

Check your answers to 2 and 3 on page 16 of this Study Guide.

C. 1. "Anthropometry, biochemical, clinical, and dietary evaluations make up the ABCD of nutrition assessment." Describe what the following components of a nutrition assessment represent. (12)

Anthropometric assessment

Biochemical (laboratory) assessment

Clinical assessment

Diet history

D. "Good nutrition and health habits can help maximize health and reduce the chances of developing nutrition-related diseases. Choices you make concerning diet, physical activity, and lifestyle all contribute to this goal." List one practice that may prevent the following ill-health outcomes. (16)

Disease condition	Preventive nutrition and health practice
High blood pressure	
Liver disease	
Anemia	
Birth defects	
Nutrient toxicities	
Obesity	
Premature heart disease	
Bone loss	
The major form of diabetes	

E. "Nutritional status is desirable for a nutrient when body tissues have enough for metabolic functions and surplus stores." Describe what the following stages of nutritional status represent in general, and then provide an example of each concept using iron storage in the body. (13)

General condition	Condition with respect to iron storage in the body
Overnutrition (toxicity)	
Desirable nutritional status	
Undernutrition	
Reduced biochemical function	
Clinical evidence	

Check your answers using Table 1-4 in your text.

F. "Food symbolizes much of what we think about ourselves." Provide two examples of this from your life while discussing the most important determinants of the foods you eat. (You listed these in the Rate Your Plate activity in Chapter 1). (20)

V. **Applying nutrition to your life**

"You will use a few mathematical concepts in studying nutrition. Besides performing addition, subtraction, multiplication, and division you need to know how to calculate percentages and convert English units of measure to metric units." The following exercise will allow you to practice math skills for nutrition. (10)

A. Jim typically has little time in the morning to prepare his favorite breakfast of an omelette, bacon, and biscuits. Instead, he usually relies on a few quick handfuls (1 ounce) of dry cereal to satisfy his hunger. Using the Table of Daily Values below (these are the nutrient standards used on food labels) and the cereal label provided, calculate the missing amounts of the specified nutrients he consumes.

Nutrient	Daily Value
vitamin C	60 milligrams
thiamin	1.5 milligrams
niacin	20 milligrams
calcium	1000 milligrams
iron	18 milligrams

Cereal Label

Nutrients	milligrams in 1 oz. of cereal	% of Daily Value	Nutrient gap
vitamin C	15 milligrams	------	------
thiamin	------	25%	75%
niacin	5 milligrams	------	------
calcium	60 milligrams	------	------
iron	------	25%	75%

B. Now practice a few metric and English conversions to fine-tune your nutrition math skills:

1 meter	=	____________	inches
1 inch	=	____________	centimeters
1 ounce	=	____________	grams
1 kilogram	=	____________	pounds
1 teaspoon	=	____________	milliliters
1 cup	=	____________	milliliters
1 cup	=	____________	tablespoons
1 quart	=	____________	cups
1 tablespoon	=	____________	teaspoons

1. A 6′2" man weighs 185 pounds. Change to centimeters and kilograms.

    ____

2. If you eat a chicken breast that is 4½ ounces, how many grams did you eat?

    ____

3. If you drank 360 milliliters of milk, how many cups did you drink?

    ____

4. A tablespoon of pureed infant food equals how many teaspoons?

    ____

5. How many quarts of milk did you drink in question 3?

    ____

Check your answers on page 16 of this Study Guide.

VI. Chapter 1 summary

This exercise will pull together the major concepts from the chapter. Fill in the blanks using the words listed at the end of this summary.

Nutrition is the study of what __________ are vital for health and how your body uses these to promote and support __________, maintenance, and __________ of cells. The nutrients in foods fall into six classes: __________, lipids (fat and oils), __________, vitamins, minerals, and ________. The first three, along with alcohol, provide __________ for the body to use. A basic plan for health promotion and disease prevention includes eating a varied diet, performing regular ______________, not smoking, limiting alcohol intake, limiting stress, and getting adequate fluid and sleep. Good nutrition should be based on eating the right foods rather than mostly relying on ______________. This strategy supplies nutrient needs and minimizes the possibility of __________. Results from large nutrition surveys in the United States suggest that some Americans need to concentrate on consuming foods that supply more vitamin A, _________, __________, iron, __________, and dietary fiber.

Our food choices are greatly affected by taste and ________, our upbringing, our ___________, and the _____ we want to present to others. There are no true junk or ______ foods. The focus should be on ___________ a total diet by choosing many __________ foods. Genetic background influences a person's risk for developing many ___________ diseases, such as obesity, heart disease, _________, and diabetes. Evidence of these diseases in one's family should make a person more attentive to avoiding "_____________" risk factors for these diseases.

Use the following words to complete the summary:

bad	culture	nutritious
balancing	energy	physical activity
calcium	foods	proteins
carbohydrates	growth	reproduction
certain B vitamins	high blood pressure	supplements
chronic	image	texture
controllable	nutrient imbalances	water
		zinc

Check your answers using the summary for Chapter 1 in your textbook; use the next page of this <u>Study Guide</u> for the last three answers.

Answers to selected questions

IV. B.2. Piña colada = (15 x 7) + (6 x 4) + (1 x 9) + (1 x 4) = 142 kcal

B.3. 1560; 38%; 46%; 15%

V. A. 25%; 75%; 0.375; 25%; 75%; 6%; 94%; 4.5

B. 39; 2.5; 28; 2.2; 5; 240; 16; 4; 3; 188/84; 126; 1.5; 3; 0.375

VI. chronic; high blood pressure; controllable

VII. Practice examination

Use this examination to test your knowledge. Cover the answers on your initial attempt.

Match the chronic disease to the possible cause:

Answer	No.	Disease	Cause
C	1.	heart disease	A. excess sodium intake
E	2.	stroke	B. long-standing alcohol intake
A	3.	high blood pressure	C. poor blood flow in the heart
D	4.	adult-onset diabetes	D. poor insulin function caused by obesity
B	5.	cirrhosis of the liver	E. blood clot in the brain

C 6. A function of carbohydrates in the diet is to:

A. absorb and transport vitamins.
B. promote growth and repair of tissues.
C. supply energy.
D. allow for enzyme action.

C 7. Good sources of carbohydrate are:

A. fats, oils, butter, and margarine.
B. fish, eggs, beef, pork, and poultry.
C. cereals, fruits, vegetables, and milk.
D. green leafy vegetables, seafood, and water.

A 8. Functions of lipids in the diet are to:

A. provide fats essential for body function.
B. transport water-soluble vitamins.
C. promote growth and repair of tissue.
D. maintain fluid balance.

A 9. Lipids are supplied in large quantities in the diet by:

A. fats, oils, meats, and nuts.
B. cereals, fruits, vegetables, and breads.
C. deep green and orange vegetables and citrus fruits.
D. green pepper, broccoli, cantaloupe, and citrus fruits.

B 10. A function of protein is to:

A. provide essential fatty acids.
B. promote growth and repair of the body.
C. make sex hormones.
D. prevent cell damage.

D 11. Good sources of protein in the diet are:

A. fats, oils, butter, and margarine.
B. green pepper, cantaloupe, citrus fruits, and broccoli.
C. deep green and orange vegetables and citrus fruits.
D. meats, fish, legumes, nuts, dairy products, and eggs.

B 12.✓ Essential nutrients:

A. are made by the body.
B. must be supplied by food.
C. include alcohol.
D. are enzymes.

B 13. A kcal is a:

A. measure of fat weight.
B. unit for expressing energy content in food.
C. scientific instrument.
D. term used to describe the amount of sugar and fat in a food.

D 14. Food likes and dislikes are affected by our senses.
In describing sensory responses to food, which term does not fit?

A. taste
B. smell
C. sight
D. nutritional value

A 15. The building blocks of proteins are:

A. amino acids.
B. fatty acids.
C. glucose units.
D. coenzymes.

C 16. Of the following the most concentrated source of energy is:

A. starch.
B. protein.
C. alcohol.
D. sugar.

C 17.✓ Which of the following is the correct number of essential nutrients for humans?

A. 5 to 10
B. 15 to 20
C. 40 to 50
D. 70 to 80

C 18.✓ The amount of fat in the human body is:

A. 13% of body weight.
B. 70% of body weight.
C. varies greatly between individuals but is often higher in women.
D. equals the weight of the muscle tissue.

D 19. To promote a nutritious diet, one should keep in mind:

A. variety.
B. moderation.
C. balance.
D. all of the above.

D 20. Which of the following would not be included in anthropometric measurements?

A. height and weight.
B. head circumference.
C. skinfold thickness.
D. blood and urine tests.

B 21. A slice of bread with 1 gram of fat, 10 grams of carbohydrate, and 2 grams of protein contains:

A. 42 kcal.
B. 57 kcal.
C. 82 kcal.
D. 102 kcal.

D 22. Nutrients that supply energy are:

A. fats and vitamins.
B. minerals and water.
C. minerals and vitamins.
D. fats and carbohydrates.

B 23. African-Americans often need to pay special attention to the amount of salt in their diet because they have a much greater chance of developing:

A. cancer.
B. high blood pressure.
C. cardiovascular disease.
D. diabetes.

D 24. A disease with a distinct genetic link is:

A. heart disease.
B. diabetes.
C. obesity.
D. all of the above.

C 25. The science of food; the nutrients and substances therein; their action, interaction, and balance in relation to health and disease is a definition of:

A. life.
B. energy metabolism.
C. nutrition.
D. food science.

Chapter 2
Tools for Diet Design

I. Points to consider

Chapter 2 is designed to allow you to:

1. Develop an eating plan based on variety, balance, and moderation.
2. Describe what the Recommended Dietary Allowances (RDAs) represent and explain why all essential nutrients do not have an RDA.
3. Describe the Food Guide Pyramid and list the nutrients that may be present in low amounts in the Guide.
4. List the Dietary Guidelines and the diseases these Guidelines are designed to prevent or minimize.
5. Compare the food groupings used in the Exchange System and the Food Guide Pyramid.
6. Describe what a nutrition label consists of and how one can be used to evaluate a food choice.

II. Word parts

Complete the following exercise using words in Chapter 2.

Word part	Meaning	Examples
is or iso	same	________
chron	time	________
chole	bile	________
osis	disease	________
scler	hard	________
vita	life	________

III. Flash cards

Cut out and review the flash cards for this chapter in Appendix A.

IV. Review and synthesis

A. 1. "You need variety in your diet because the required nutrients are scattered among many different foods." Complete the Food Guide Pyramid summary based on adult recommendations. (40-41)

Food Group	Servings	Major Nutrients	Examples of Food Choices
Milk, yogurt, and cheese			milk, cheese, yogurt, cottage cheese, custard/pudding, and ice cream
Meat, poultry, fish, dry beans, eggs, and nuts			cooked meat, poultry, fish, cooked dry beans, and eggs
Fruits			cooked fruit, fruit juices, fresh fruits, and salads
Vegetables			raw vegetables, cooked vegetables, and vegetable juices
Breads, cereals, rice, and pasta			bread, ready-to-eat cereal, cooked cereal, rice, and pasta
Fats, oils, and sweets			margarine, vegetable oil, and candy bars

2. "The foundations of nutrition are variety, balance, and moderation." Describe how to use the Food Guide Pyramid. What are two of its strengths and two of its weaknesses? (39)

B. 1. "The Food Guide Pyramid was designed to help meet nutritional needs for carbohydrate, protein, fat, vitamins, and minerals. However, most of the major chronic 'killer' diseases in America, such as heart disease, cancer, and alcoholism, are not primarily associated with deficiencies of these nutrients." List the Dietary Guidelines for Americans. Next to each Guideline note a specific disease being addressed. (46)

a.

b.

c.

d.

e.

f.

g.

2. Why is this type of nutrition education important if there is enough food for us to buy?

C. "The healthy eating habits that result from implementing the Food Guide Pyramid and Dietary Guidelines can pay you lifelong dividends in good health." Table 2-5 gives some advice for applying dietary guidelines to one's own diet. Practice alternating some food habits you want to change by substituting more healthful options. (48)

Your typical food choices	A more healthful option
1.	
2.	
3.	
4.	
5.	

D. 1. "Thus the RDAs are estimates of the amount of each nutrient that should be consumed by healthy people to meet their nutritional needs." How should the RDAs be generally applied when evaluating human dietary intakes? (52)

If your dietary intake is less than the RDA for a nutrient, do you necessarily have a deficient diet? Why? (52)

2. "Estimated safe and adequate daily dietary intakes (ESADDI) have been established for several nutrients. The Board determined that insufficient data were available to set RDAs." List four vitamins and/or minerals for which only estimated safe and adequate intakes have been established. (53 and inside cover of textbook)

a. c.

b. d.

E. "When setting the RDA for children, scientists add extra protein to create the positive balance necessary to accommodate daily growth needs in new cells." The RDA for protein for adults is 0.8 grams per kilogram of one's healthy body weight. (Remember 1 kilogram = 2.2 pounds). Complete the following exercise in relation to protein needed for a 42-year-old man who weighs 172 pounds. (52)

Persons' RDA for protein:

Possible protein food sources:

Symptoms of protein deficiency:

When would this man be (or have been) in the following states of health?

positive protein balance

protein equilibrium

negative protein balance

Check your numerical answers on page 30 in this Study Guide.

F. 1. "The Food and Drug Administration (FDA) has developed a set of generic standards, called *Daily Values*, that are used to express the nutrient content of foods for the Nutrition Facts panel on food labels." Compare the RDA and the Daily Values for your age and gender for vitamin A, vitamin E, calcium, and iron. Which of these RDA are quite different than the Daily Values? (See the inside cover and Appendix C in your textbook.) (54)

a. vitamin A

b. vitamin E

c. calcium

d. iron

2. What are the Reference Daily Intakes (RDIs), and on what are they based? How do they relate to the Daily Values? (55)

3. Daily Reference Values (DRVs) serve what purpose? How do they relate to Daily Values? (55)

G. Describe briefly how the Exchange System differs from the Food Guide Pyramid and the Dietary Guidelines in terms of a tool for diet planning. (57)

V. Applying nutrition to your life

"Foods packaged and sold in the United States are labeled." Answer the following questions about "Wheat and Raisins" based on the label. (64)

"WHEAT AND RAISINS"

NUTRITION FACTS
Serving Size 3/4 cup (24 g)
Servings Per Container 18

AMOUNT PER SERVING
Calories 110 Calories from Fat 9%

	% Daily Value
Total Fat 1 g	2%
Saturated Fat 0.5 g	3%
Cholesterol 0 mg	0%
Sodium 140 mg	6%
Total Carbohydrate 23 g	8%
Sugars 5 g	
Dietary Fiber 3 g	12%
Protein 2 g	

Briefly explain what Daily Value represents in everyday terms.

Vitamin A 25% Vitamin C 2% Calcium 4%
Iron 25%

Why are only a few vitamins and minerals listed? Are the others simply not present?

*Percents (%) of a Daily Value are based on a 2,000 calorie diet. Your Daily Values may vary higher or lower depending on your calorie needs:

Nutrient		2,000 Calories	2,500 Calories
Total Fat	Less than	65g	80g
Sat Fat	Less than	20g	25g
Cholesterol	Less than	300 mg	300 mg
Sodium	Less than	2,400 mg	2,400 mg
Total Carbohydrate		300g	375g
Fiber		25g	30g

Many of the Daily Values are based on Daily Reference Values (DRVs). What do the DRV's represent? Are they the same as RDAs?

INGREDIENTS:
Whole wheat, raisins, sugar, honey, brown sugar syrup, salt, cereal malt syrup, calcium carbonate, trisodium phosphate, a B vitamin (niacinamide), iron (a mineral nutrient), annatto extract color, vitamin A (palmitate), vitamin B-6 (pyridoxine hydrochloride), vitamin B-2 (riboflavin), vitamin B-1 (thiamin mononitrate), A B vitamin (folic acid).

What ingredient is in the greatest amount based on weight?

How many forms of sweeteners are in this product?

CAPTAIN MILLS, INC.
ST. PAUL, MINNESOTA 55440
Made in U.S.A.

Where could you write to find more information about this product or file a complaint?

VI. Chapter 2 summary

Fill in the blanks using the words listed at the end of this summary.

The Food Guide Pyramid is designed to translate nutrient recommendations into a food plan that exhibits _________, balance, and _________ while focusing on choosing _________ (or nonfat) dairy products and some vegetable _________, in addition to animal protein foods, citrus fruits, and dark green vegetables, and emphasizing ___________ breads and cereals.

Dietary guidelines have been issued to help reduce __________ "killer" diseases. The guidelines emphasize eating a _________ of foods; maintaining healthy body weight; moderating consumption of _________, cholesterol, sugar, _________, and _________; and eating plenty of fruits, vegetables, and grain products.

Recommended Dietary Allowances are set for many nutrients. These amounts yield enough of each nutrient to meet the needs for essentially all groups of _________ people within specific _________ and _________ groups.

Daily Values are used as a basis for expressing the nutrient content of _________ on the Nutrition Facts panel. Reference Daily Intakes (RDIs), which are derived from the _________ values, constitute the majority of the Daily Values. Daily Reference Values (DRVs) have been set for some nutrients with no ______, such as fat and ______; they comprise the rest of the _______.

Another diet planning system, the __________, provides a powerful tool for estimating the carbohydrate, fat, protein, and energy content of a food or meal and for planning a diet to correspond to specific goals for _________, fat, protein, and _________ consumption.

Foods packaged and sold in any United States supermarket usually are labeled with the ______, the manufacturer's name and address, the amount of product in the package, and the _________ listed in order of amount from most to least by _________. Since the early 1990s, most manufacturers also must add a _________ panel. This lists the serving size of the product, the number of servings per package, and many nutrient amounts per serving based on the ______.

Use the following words to complete the summary:

age	fats	product name
alcohol	foods	proteins
carbohydrate	gender	RDA
chronic	healthy	salt
Daily Values (DVs) (2x)	ingredients	variety (2x)
dietary fiber	low-fat	weight
energy	moderation	whole grain
Exchange System	Nutrition Facts	1968 RDA

Check your answers using the summary for Chapter 2 in your textbook; use page 30 of this Study Guide for the last five answers.

VII. Practice examination

Cover the answers on your initial attempt.

A 1. The RDA are nutrient quantities:

A. used as guidelines for diet planning for groups.
B. that ensure good health for all individuals.
C. that represent minimum daily needs.
D. all of the above.

B 2. If your daily intake of a vitamin does not meet the RDA:

A. you necessarily have a poor diet.
B. you may not be meeting your needs.
C. this is of no consequence because the RDA are designed for groups.
D. you are safe if you meet at least half the RDA.

D 3. A Nutrition Facts panel listing selected vitamin and mineral contents must appear:

A. if a vitamin or mineral has been lost in processing.
B. only if the manufacturer advertises the nutritional benefits for the food.
C. if the food uses "enriched" flour.
D. on almost all foods.

A 4. "Enriched" grains do NOT have which one of the following substances added back?

A. dietary fiber
B. niacin
C. iron
D. thiamin

D 5. One of the following is NOT a U.S. Dietary Guideline?

A. maintain a healthy body weight.
B. moderate sugar use.
C. moderate sodium use.
D. moderate starch use.

D 6. The RDA stands for:

A. recommended daily allowance.
B. required dietary allowance.
C. required daily allowance.
D. recommended dietary allowance.

D 7. The basic message of nutrition is:

A. variety.
B. moderation.
C. balance.
D. all of the above.

D 8. Labeling laws require that ingredients in food products be listed on the container in descending order of their:

A. kilocalories.
B. cost.
C. nutrient density.
D. weight.

A 9. An estimated safe and adequate daily dietary allowance:

A. is set for some nutrients instead of an RDA.
B. gives a range for the RDA.
C. is used to set the U.S. RDA.
D. reflects weekly needs.

B 10. The adult U.S. RDA:

A. is designed specifically for Americans, whereas the RDA applies to all people.
B. generally represents the highest nutrient needs in the "adult" RDA category.
C. includes all nutrients.
D. applies to individuals, whereas the RDA applies to groups.

B 11. Which suggestion would NOT greatly improve the possible nutrient "weaknesses" of the Food Guide Pyramid?

A. use whole grains.
B. double milk portions.
C. eat more broccoli.
D. eat more kidney beans.

C 12. Dietary Guidelines have been issued primarily to decrease:

A. vitamin E deficiencies in the United States.
B. weaknesses in the Food Guide Pyramid.
C. the incidence of chronic "killer" diseases.
D. weaknesses in the RDA.

C 13. Food choices in the Exchange System are grouped according to similarities in _________ content.

A. kcalorie, carbohydrate, fat, and vitamin.
B. kcalorie, protein, fat, and vitamin.
C. kcalorie, protein, fat, and carbohydrate.
D. vitamin, mineral, and water.

B 14. Substituting beans and seeds for meats and using whole-grain instead of refined breads and cereals improves the nutrient content of the diet by increasing intake of:

A. vitamins A, D, and C and calcium.
B. magnesium, vitamin E, vitamin B-6, iron, and zinc.
C. thiamin, calcium, and vitamin D.
D. vitamins B-12 and K, chloride, and magnesium.

D 15. The Food Guide Pyramid provides the full allowance of:

A. all essential nutrients.
B. all essential nutrients except energy.
C. most of the essential nutrients, along with energy.
D. most of the essential nutrients, except energy, for many people.

A 16. The RDA for energy are based on:

A. average needs.
B. average needs plus a 30% margin of safety.
C. 90% of average needs.
D. double the minimum requirement.

Match the following words with the definitions below.

18 sugar free	24 cholesterol free	23 fortified
19 low cholesterol	20 low calorie	21 enriched
17 very low sodium	22 good source	25 low sodium

17. The product contains no more than 35 milligrams of sodium per serving.

18. The product contains less than 0.5 grams of sugar per serving.

19. The product contains 20 milligrams or less of cholesterol and 2 grams or less of saturated fat per serving.

20. The product contains no more than 40 kcal per serving.

21. The vitamins thiamin, riboflavin, and niacin and the mineral iron have been added to the product to replace what is lost in processing.

22. The food contains 10% to 19% of the Daily Value for a particular nutrient.

23. Vitamins and/or minerals that were not originally present have been added to the product.

24. The product contains less than 2 milligrams of cholesterol and less than 2 grams of saturated fat per serving.

25. The product contains no more than 140 milligrams of sodium per serving.

Answers to selected chapter questions

IV. B. $\frac{172}{2.2} = 78.2$ kg

$78.2 \times 0.8 = 62.6$ grams protein for RDA

VI. product name; ingredients; weight; Nutrition Facts; Daily Values

---

Chapter 3
Nutritional Advice: Facts and Fallacies

I. Points to consider

Chapter 3 is designed to allow you to:

1. Identify sources of nutrition quackery.
2. Understand the basis of the scientific method as it is used in developing hypotheses and theories in the field of nutrition.
3. Compare the nutritional quality and safety of organically grown foods with those of conventionally grown foods.
4. Compare and contrast nutritional quality and safety of "health" foods with those of typical foods in a grocery store.
5. Identify characteristics of meganutrient therapy, herbal therapy, and macrobiotics.
6. Evaluate the pros and cons of use of vitamin and mineral supplements.

II. Word parts

Complete the following exercise using words in Chapter 3.

Word part	Meaning	Examples
quack	impostor	______________
organic	pertaining to the body, living	______________
mega	big, great	______________
macro	large, long	______________
syn	with, together	______________
-icide	to kill	______________
herb	leafy plant	______________

III. Flash cards

Cut out and review the flash cards for this chapter in Appendix A.

IV. **Review and synthesis**

A. "This approach also reduces the chance that the subjects may begin to feel better simply because they are participating in a research study or receiving a new treatment." Design a simple double-blind study to test whether high doses of vitamin C cure baldness. (77)

Check your answer on page 40 of this Study Guide.

B. "Advocates of organic foods claim these crops offer more nutrition and fewer health hazards than conventionally grown foods." Compare and contrast claims made by organic gardeners with the findings of nutrition scientists. (89-90)

(HINT: Compare their views on pesticides, fertilizers, and nutritional quality of foods.)

Claims of "organic" gardeners	versus	Findings of nutrition scientists

C. 1. "Food manufacturers add preservatives and other additives to many products. The controversy surrounding use of additives is largely groundless in view of their usefulness and safety." List two pros and cons for use of food additives. (91)

	Pros	Cons
a.		
b.		

2. "Although it is illegal for storekeepers to diagnose or prescribe, they often do both. No special knowledge or training is required to become a salesperson at a health food store." Review Table 3-1; have you ever been a victim of any of these claims? Were they beneficial in your opinion? (73)

D. 1. "Telling the difference between a reputable and a bogus organization is not always easy, even for health care professionals." The chapter cautions you to beware of misinformation. List three phrases that should warn you to proceed with caution. (98)

a.

b.

c.

2. "If you suspect false claims about a product or service, seek answers from reputable sources." The chapter offers some suggestions for reliable sources of nutrition information. Name four below. (98 and Table 3-2)

a.

b.

c.

d.

E. "People tend to believe what they hear repeatedly. As with any type of brainwashing, a repeated claim can seem real even when it has no basis in fact. Unsound nutritional claims flood the media, food shelves, and conversations of those seeking good health." Design your own venture to promote a "quack" product or service, then verbally promote the claim to family and friends. Note their reactions. (74)

Did they believe you?

What questions did they ask?

Was there a common characteristic among those who believed you? Why is this important?

F. "Nutrition scientists generally agree that most people can obtain the vitamins and minerals they need if they eat a healthy diet. If you eat a balanced, low-fat, varied diet that conforms to the Food Guide Pyramid and engage in regular physical activity, you probably don't need supplements." List four conditions for which supplementation may be recommended as suggested by the American Institute of Nutrition and the American Society for Clinical Nutrition. (105)

a.

b.

c.

d.

V. Applying nutrition to your life

"Health food retailers often suggest remedies for illnesses best treated by a medical professional. Protect yourself by being an informed and skeptical consumer."

Is the health food store all it's cracked up to be? Many people believe that health food stores are a better place to buy certain foods and supplements than conventional markets. However, identical product brands are often found in both types of stores. In this assignment you are asked to do a price comparison of foods in a health-food store and those in a conventional market.

1. Go to the local health-food store and pick six food items that you think would be sold at a conventional market. Pick plain items like raisins, brown rice, honey, and kidney beans. Also note the type of supplements available in health-food stores. Does it surprise you that people feel the need to purchase and use many of these products?

2. Record the price and weight of the six food items.

3. Calculate the price per pound or ounce.
   Example: a 12-ounce jar of honey costs $3.48.
   $3.48 / 12 ounces = $.29 per ounce

4. Find the same items in a conventional supermarket.

5. Do steps 2 and 3 above for these products.

6. Compare these products based on price per amount (as in pound or ounce).
   Are the prices consistently higher at the health-food store than at the conventional market? If so, do you see any reason why the products should be more expensive?

VI. Chapter 3 summary

Fill in the blanks using the words listed at the end of this summary.

The _________ method is a logical approach for determining the accuracy of _________ ("educated guesses"). A _________ study is the gold standard for experimental work because it reduces the potential for ___________ introduced by the investigators, subjects, and especially the ________ effect.

Though capable of causing bodily harm, _________ hits hardest in the pocketbook. Abandoning medical therapy for quack cures may result in serious _________ consequences.

_________ and so-called health foods provide alternatives to foods containing artificial ingredients and _________ and to foods grown with chemical fertilizers and _________. But the overall health and nutritional benefits are few if any.

Quacks often suggest that the average diet lacks _________ and minerals and so should be supplemented with their products. Choosing whole grains, fruits, and vegetables and other selections from the _________ provides excellent nutrition. An excess of certain vitamins and minerals, such as vitamins A and D and the minerals iron and copper, can cause __________.

_________ remedies and megadose vitamin and mineral therapies are not necessarily reliable and may be _________.

Consumers feeling short-changed by conventional health care provide a large and willing market for those promoting questionable and dangerous nutritional advice. Before "accepting" alternative health products or suggestions, check for supporting evidence and _________. If in doubt, check with a _________ or Registered Dietitian.

Any new recommendation for changes in diet habits should be evaluated by using _______ that can either support or refute the recommendation. The health of nutrition science is fostered by a _______ that does not accept a hypothesis as "fact" until manifest proof is available. With regard to supplements, the Council on Scientific Affairs of the American Medical Association recommends that a supplement contain no more than _________ of the adult ___________. A balanced supplement formulation conforming to these guidelines minimizes the chance of vitamin

and mineral ________, ________, and other undesirable effects.

Use the following words to complete the summary:

additives	herbal	reputable credentials
bias	hypotheses	rigorous experiments
competition	organically grown	scientific
Daily Values	pesticides	skeptical mind
dangerous	physician	toxicity
double-blind	physical	vitamins
Food Guide Pyramid	placebo	50% to 150%
harm	quackery	

Check your answers using the summary for Chapter 3 in your textbook; use page 40 for the final six answers.

VII. Practice examination

Cover the answers on your initial attempt.

C 1. Americans spend over _________ dollars a year on health fraud.

A. 3 billion
B. 70 billion
C. 30 billion
D. 125 billion

B 2. One group which seems particularly vulnerable to quackery is:

A. mothers.
B. elderly persons.
C. teenagers.
D. religious persons.

A 3. Who is ultimately responsible for protecting you from false advertising and misleading health claims?

A. yourself
B. doctors
C. government
D. radio, television, and newspaper executives

B 4. Organically grown foods are much safer and provide better nutrient quality than conventionally grown foods.

A. True
B. False

B 5. Which of the following terms typically would not be used to define the word natural?

A. minimal processing
B. recycled
C. no additives
D. no artificial ingredients

D 6. Grains such as wheat and rice provide many nutrients. However, there is one part of the grain that is indigestible and must be stripped away. This is known as the:

A. gum.
B. starch.
C. bran.
D. hull.

D 7. Which of the following functions is an additive capable of doing?

A. preventing off flavors
B. enhancing nutrient value
C. retaining food crispness
D. all of the above

A 8. Which of the following is a typical characteristic of foods in a health food store?

A. they cost more.
B. these are foods we need that cannot be found elsewhere.
C. the food contains extra nutrients.
D. the food is always fresh.

B 9. It is a proven fact that stress raises vitamin needs.

A. True.
B. False.

B 10. The terms willow bark, sarsaparilla, comfrey, and senna are all names of:

A. pesticides.
B. herbal products.
C. sources of meganutrients.
D. synthetic drugs.

D 11. Which of the following most accurately defines herbs?

A. contain magical properties
B. useful medicines
C. completely safe
D. necessitate caution and medical guidance with use

C 12. Macrobiotics, originated by philosopher George Ohsawa, originally emphasized a diet rich in:

A. foods of animal origin.
B. whole grain and soybean products.
C. vegetables and brown rice.
D. nuts and seeds.

B 13. In former and current macrobiotic diets, one important type of food that is often missing is:

A. whole grains.
B. milk products.
C. vegetables.
D. sweets.

D 14. The American Association of Nutrition Consultants and the International Academy of Nutrition Consultants both:

A. are highly rated professional organizations of nutrition science.
B. give advance training in nutrition consulting.
C. are elite groups of nutrition experts.
D. are places where one can purchase degrees.

D 15. Which of the following has (have) been known to provide misleading nutritional information:

A. Nutritional Health Federation.
B. health food stores.
C. chiropractors.
D. all of the above.

A 16. A safe standard of one's RDA is to meet a least 70%. Keep in mind, however, that some nutrients are potentially toxic at high doses. So it is best not to exceed _________ of the Daily Values unless under medical supervision.

A. 150%
B. 200%
C. 500%
D. 1000%

A 17. Epidemiological studies yield nutrition information through:

A. correlations of diets with disease in certain populations.
B. study of archaeological findings.
C. laboratory experiments.
D. chemical analysis of foods.

B 18. When scientists observe occurrences that cannot be explained, they attempt to formulate questions that may provide possible explanations for the phenomena. Another name for these questions are:

A. theories.
B. hypotheses.
C. experiments.
D. placebos

E 19. Quackery can significantly harm or kill its victims by:

A. promoting unsafe or hazardous products.
B. delaying effective treatment for serious conditions.
C. abandoning effective treatment.
D. impoverishment; victims being harmed economically.
E. A, B, and C.

D 20. A double-blind study:

A. uses blind subjects.
B. is required in all research.
C. may omit controls to reduce experimental costs.
D. uses a placebo.

D 21. Potentially toxic herbs include:

A. hai gen fen
B. jin bu huan
C. chaparral
D. all of the above

B 22. Most scientific discoveries are made in a miraculous flash.

A. True
B. False

A 23. Comparing individuals who have the condition in question, such as lung cancer, with individuals who do not have the condition, is part of a:

A. case-control study.
B. double-blind study.
C. experimental study.
D. epidemiological study.

D 24. Bogus health claims generally use which of the following for support?

A. testimonials about personal experience
B. dramatic results (rarely true)
C. extreme bias against the medical community or traditional medical treatments
D. all of the above

A 25. The terms organic and inorganic, based on chemical concepts, also are used to describe certain types of farming methods.

A. True
B. False

Answers to selected questions

IV. A. Double-blind study: Find 20 bald men. Give 10 men a high dose of vitamin C each day for a month while the other 10 men receive a placebo ("fake medicine"). Neither the subjects nor you can know who receives which treatment. Your friend holds the code and only divulges it after the experiment ends and any new hair growth is documented.

VI. rigorous experiments; skeptical mind; 50% to 150%; Daily Values; competition; toxicity

---

Chapter 4
The Human Body: A Nutrition Perspective

I. Points to consider

Chapter 4 is designed to allow you to:

1. Outline the organs used in digestion and absorption.
2. Describe the function of each organ used in the digestive process and the flow of the process.
3. Become familiar with the enzyme classes that act on each nutrient group.
4. Describe the processes used for food absorption into the body.
5. Outline the role of the heart, kidneys, nerves, muscles, hormones, and hormone-like factors in digestion and absorption.
6. Identify some conditions that result when digestive processes are hampered.

II. Word parts

Complete the following exercise using words in Chapter 4.

Word part	Meaning	Examples
gastr	stomach	________________
zym	ferment	________________
aut	self	________________
phag	eat	________________
hepat	liver	________________
peps	digest	________________
ase	enzyme	________________

III. Flash cards

Cut out and review the flash cards for this chapter in Appendix A.

IV. Review and synthesis

A. 1. "Often two or more tissues combine to form more complex organs." Briefly define the following terms. (112)

a. cell

b. tissue

c. organ

d. organ system (e.g. bone)

2. "Although most cells in our bodies contain the same DNA information, each cell is programmed to use only the parts of the DNA instructions that apply to its own tasks." Describe how DNA allows for the development of different cells, and in doing so, for different organ systems. (112)

B. "At still higher levels of coordination, several organs can cooperate to achieve a common purpose and form an organ system." Describe the roles the following organ systems play in the nutritional processes and overall health of the body. (113)

a. cardiovascular system

b. endocrine system

c. nervous system

d. digestive system

e. immune system

f. storage system (e.g. adipose cells)

C. "The hormone insulin helps control the amount of glucose in the blood, and thyroid hormones help control the body's metabolic rate. Other hormones are especially important in regulating digestive processes, such as the hormone gastrin, which is produced in the stomach." Complete the descriptions of the secretions and products of the digestive tract. (116)

Secretion	Site of production	Purpose
Saliva		Contributes to starch digestion, lubrication
Mucus	Mouth, stomach, small intestine, large intestine	
	Mouth, stomach, small intestine, pancreas	Promote digestion of foodstuffs into particles small enough for absorption
Acid	Stomach	
Bile		Suspends fat in water to aid fat digestion in the small intestine
	Pancreas	Neutralizes stomach acid when it reaches the small intestine
Hormones	Stomach, small intestine	

D. "The circulatory system distributes nutrients yielded from digestion and absorption, along with oxygen from the air, to all body cells. All blood goes to the lungs to pick up oxygen and release carbon dioxide. The oxygenated blood then returns to the heart to be pumped to all other body tissues." Describe what takes place with respect to the circulatory system in the following organs. (115)

a. lungs

b. heart

c. small intestine

d. liver

e. lower extremities

E. "Fluids and particles leaving the villi in the intestine drain into two different circulation systems." Classify each term in the box with the expected transport system. (114)

Portal vein	Lymphatic vessels
____________	____________
____________	____________
____________	
____________	
____________	

alcohol
amino acids
fat-soluble vitamins
minerals
monosaccharides
triglycerides (long-chain)
water-soluble vitamins

Check your answers on page 52 in this Study Guide.

F. "Each type of enzyme can speed only one specific type of chemical process. For example, enzymes that recognize and digest table sugar ignore milk sugar (lactose)." Malabsorption of lactose, as you will further research in Chapter 5, may cause bloating, diarrhea, flatus, and abdominal discomfort. Why? (122, 127)

G. 1. "The small intestine absorbs nutrients through various means." What is active absorption? (124)

Why is it necessary for glucose?

2. Describe the two other main types of absorption.

H. "The presence of feces in the rectum stimulates elimination." What are two functions of the large intestine? (127)

a.

b.

I. "People with ulcers should also refrain from smoking and minimize the use of aspirin and other related compounds." Provide some dietary and other practical advice for people who suffer from the following disorders: (135)

a. ulcers

b. heartburn

c. constipation

d. hemorrhoids

e. irritable bowel syndrome

V. Applying nutrition to your life

"The gastrointestinal tract is also known as the alimentary canal." Label each part indicated in the figure using the following terms, and briefly describe each part's role, if any, in digestion and absorption. Check your answers using Figure 4-3 in your textbook.

---

pancreas, anus, trachea, salivary glands, appendix, mouth, esophagus, large intestine (colon) (2x), liver, rectum, stomach, small intestine, epiglottis, gallbladder, pyloric sphincter, common bile duct

---

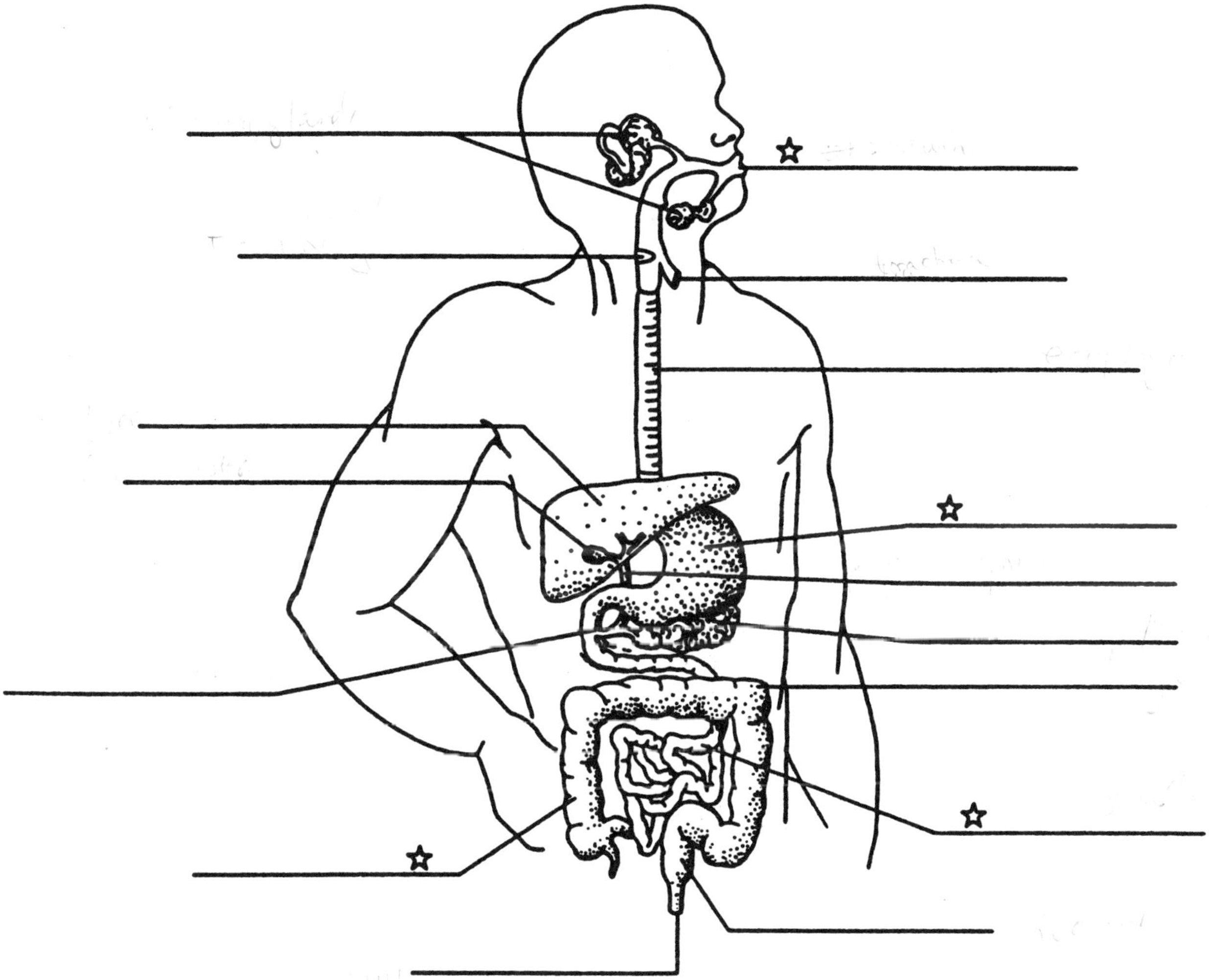

VI. Chapter 4 summary

Fill in the blanks using the words listed at the end of this summary.

The __________ is the basic building block of body tissues. __________ is the blueprint found in all cells. It determines the cell type as it is used to produce specific ________ and ________ for each type of cell. Blood travels the _________ in which oxygen is picked up by the lungs. The systemic circuit delivers essential nutrients, energy, _________, and water to all body cells. Nutrients and wastes are exchanged between the blood and the cell across the _________. Water-soluble compounds in the _________ enter the _________ and travel to the liver. Fat-soluble compounds enter into the _________, which eventually connects to the _________.

The ____________ consists of the mouth, _________, stomach, _________, large intestine (colon), rectum, and anus. For the most part, digestion and _________ of nutrients occurs in the small intestine. The _________, gallbladder, and _________ participate in digestion and absorption. Products from these organs, such as _________ and bile, enter the small intestine and play important roles in digesting protein, fat, and ________. Along the GI tract are ringlike ________ that control the flow of foodstuffs. Muscular contractions called _________ propel the foodstuffs down the GI tract. A variety of nerves, hormones, and other substances control the process.

Digestive enzymes are secreted by the mouth, _________, and wall of the _________ intestine and pancreas. The presence of food in the small intestine stimulates the release of pancreatic enzymes. _________ needed for ________ digestion is synthesized by the liver, stored in the _______, and released in digestion. The major absorptive sites consist of fingerlike projections called villi in the small intestine. _________ cover the villi. Most digestion and absorption occurs in the small intestine. Little digestion or absorption occurs in either the stomach or _________ intestine. Some _________ are digested in the stomach. Some plant fibers are digested by the _________ present in the _________. Final ______ and mineral absorption takes place in the large intestine. The presence of _________ in the _________ provides a strong impetus for elimination.

The kidneys, __________, and lungs all perform excretory functions for the body. Limited stores of ________ are present in the blood for immediate use and stored to a greater or lesser extent in body tissues for later use when sufficient food is unavailable.

A person who is prone to developing ulcers should not _________. Minimizing the use of __________ also is important because of its resulting irritation to the stomach. This combination of therapies, along with the use of antibiotics and antacid medications, has revolutionized ulcer therapy. An important dietary measure for avoiding heartburn is to eat ________ meals low in fat. Meals containing much fat remain in the stomach longer and create pressure in the stomach that can force stomach ________ into the esophagus. Adequate _________, physical activity, and _________ are important for preventing constipation.

Use the following words to complete the summary:

absorption
absorptive cells
acid
aspirin
bacteria
bile
bloodstream
carbohydrate
cell
cell membrane
chemicals
dietary fiber
DNA
enzymes
esophagus

fat
feces
fluid
gallbladder
gastrointestinal
(GI) tract
large
large intestine
liver
lymphatic system
nutrients
oxygen
pancreas
peristalsis
proteins

portal vein
pulmonary circuit
rectum
skin
small
smaller
small intestine
smoke
stomach
structures
triglyceride
valves
(sphincters)
villi
water

Check your answers using the summary for Chapter 4 in your textbook; use page 52 of this Study Guide for the last six answers.

VII. Practice examination

Cover the answers on your initial attempt.

B 1. The best treatment for an ulcer is the milk and cream therapy.

A. True
B. False

C 2. The liver is the first stop for most absorbed nutrients because it:

A. lies so close to the intestine.
B. controls blood flow to the heart.
C. is the end point for the portal vein.
D. must respond by making the correct amount of insulin.

C 3. The major site for fluid absorption in the gastrointestinal tract is the:

A. esophagus.
B. stomach.
C. small intestine.
D. colon.

D 4. The gnawing pain in the upper chest that is caused by acid flowing back into the esophagus from the stomach is termed:

A. lactose intolerance.
B. ulcer.
C. hemorrhoids.
D. heartburn.

C 5. The function of mucus in the stomach is to:

A. neutralize stomach acid.
B. activate pepsinogen to form pepsin.
C. protect stomach cells from autodigestion.
D. emulsify fats.

D 6. The pyloric sphincter:

A. prevents the contents of the intestine from backing up into the stomach.
B. secretes acid into the stomach.
C. holds the food in the stomach long enough for it to be thoroughly mixed and liquefied.
D. A and C.

C 7. A sensible idea for preventing constipation is to:

A. use a laxative when needed.
B. cut down on water intake.
C. include more high-fiber foods in the diet.
D. include fewer high-fiber foods in the diet.

C 8. The lining of the gastrointestinal tract is replaced completely about every:

A. 12 hours.
B. day.
C. 2 to 5 days.
D. 2 weeks.

D 9. Nutrient(s) that support immune function include

A. vitamin A
B. vitamin B-6
C. zinc
D. all of the above

__C__ 10. Nutrients that enter the lymph for absorption are:

A. ascorbic acid, minerals, amino acids, and cholesterol.
B. short-chain fatty acids, triglycerides, and cholesterol.
C. long-chain fatty acids, triglycerides, and vitamin A.
D. minerals, short-chain fatty acids, and carotenoids.

__D__ 11. Much of the digestion that occurs in the large intestine is caused by:

A. lipase.
B. pepsin.
C. saliva.
D. bacteria.

Match the following:

__C__ 12. peristalsis
__I__ 13. sphincter
__H__ 14. chyme
__A__ 15. mucus
__G__ 16. tissue
__E__ 17. epiglottis
__F__ 18. colon
__B__ 19. active absorption
__E__ 20. passive absorption

A. Acts as a lubricant and protein for stomach cells
B. Transport system requiring that energy be expended by the cell to pump a compound into the cell
C. Muscle contractions of the gut
D. Molecules cross cell membranes without use of carrier molecules or energy expenditure
E. Closes off the trachea during swallowing to prevent food from entering the lungs
F. Reabsorbs water from undigested food and waste materials
G. A group of cells designed to perform a specific function
H. A mixture of stomach secretions and partially digested foods
I. A muscular valve that controls flow of food stuff

__B__ 21. The portal vein:

A. carries blood from the lungs to the heart.
B. collects blood from the intestinal capillary bed and carries it to the liver.
C. delivers fat and soluble compounds to the lymphatic system.
D. is also known as the alimentary canal.

__D__ 22. Short-term storage of carbohydrate occurs:

A. in the intestinal mucosa.
B. when the skin is exposed to the sun.
C. as amino acid reserves in the bloodstream.
D. in the muscle and liver.

__C__ 23. Bile is formed in the:

A. pancreas.
B. walls of the small intestine.
C. liver.
D. gallbladder.

__A__ 24. Digestion begins in the:

A. mouth.
B. stomach.
C. small intestine.
D. pancreas.

__A__ 25. Although irritable bowel syndrome can be uncomfortable and upsetting, it is harmless; it carries no risk for cancer or other serious digestive problems.

A. True
B. False

Answers to selected questions

IV. D.	portal vein	alcohol, amino acids, minerals, monosaccharides, water-soluble vitamins
	lymphatic vessels	fat-soluble vitamins, triglycerides (long-chain)
VI.	smoke; aspirin; smaller; acid; dietary fiber; fluid	

Chapter 5
Carbohydrates

I. Points to consider

Chapter 5 is designed to allow you to:

1. Relate the major carbohydrates, which are monosaccharides, disaccharides, polysaccharides, and dietary fiber, in terms of their basic structures and food sources.
2. List the functions of carbohydrate in the body and the problems that result from not eating enough.
3. Describe the regulation of blood glucose and the nutrients that can become blood glucose.
4. Outline the effects of dietary fiber on the body.
5. List guidelines for carbohydrate intake.
6. Describe food sources of carbohydrate and list some alternate sweeteners.
7. Identify the consequences of lactose intolerance and diabetes, and appropriate dietary measures to take to reduce these health problems.

II. Word parts

Complete the following exercise using words in Chapter 5.

Word part	Meaning	Examples
mono	one	________________
poly	many	________________
ose	sugar	________________
glyc	glucose	________________
hyper	over, above	________________
hypo	under	________________
sacchar	sugar	________________

III. **Flash cards**

Cut out and review the flash cards for this chapter in Appendix A.

IV. **Review and synthesis**

A. "Saliva contains an enzyme called salivary amylase. This enzyme breaks down starch into many smaller sugar units (disaccharides such as maltose)." Describe the digestion of a breakfast, consisting of a glass of grape juice, a slice of toast with jelly, and a bowl of cereal and milk by indicating the part of the digestive tract where each of the following occur. (145-146)

1. ______ The disaccharides, sucrose (in the jelly), and lactose (in the milk) are broken down by enzymes into their respective monosaccharides.

2. ______ Starch (in the bread and cereal) is broken down by the enzyme salivary amylase.

3. ______ Starch and its partial breakdown products are broken down to maltose by the enzyme pancreatic amylase.

4. ______ Salivary amylase is inactivated by strong acid. The digestion of starch is then temporarily halted.

5. ______ Absorption of glucose, fructose (from the grape juice), and galactose (from the milk sugar) takes place.

B. 1. "The main function of glucose is to supply energy for the body. Certain tissues in the body, such as red blood cells, can use only this and other simple carbohydrate forms for energy." Describe briefly three functions of carbohydrates. (147)

a.

b.

c.

2. "Under normal circumstances, a person's blood glucose concentration is regulated within a very narrow range." The hormones that regulate blood glucose include: (149)

a.

b.

c.

Briefly note the effects of each on blood glucose.

3. "On the tip of the tongue are sensors for tasting sweetness." Rank these sugars in order of sweetness. (150)

maltose, sucrose, glucose, fructose, sorbitol

How does the sweetness of aspartame compare to these sugars?

4. "If you don't eat enough carbohydrates, your body is forced to make glucose from other nutrients." Briefly describe what medical problems are associated with a low-carbohydrate diet. (Hint: what happens to protein and other body constituents when carbohydrates cannot be used as an energy source?) (151)

a.

b.

C. 1. "Dietary fiber is not a single substance but a group of substances with similar characteristics." Complete this table on the classification of dietary fibers. (144)

Type	Component	Examples	Physiological effects	Major food sources
Insoluble				
Noncarbohydrate	______	______	Under study	All plants
Carbohydrate	Cellulose	______	Increases fecal bulk	______
	______	Brown rice	Decreases transit time	Wheat, ______, ______, ______
Soluble				
Carbohydrate	______, gums, ______, ______	Apples, ______, ______, carrots, barley, ______, ______	Delays gastric emptying; slows glucose absorption; ______	______, oat products, ______

2. "When enough fiber is consumed, its water-retaining property helps enlarge and soften the stool, easing elimination." List two potential benefits of fiber in the diet. (152)

a.

b.

D. 1. "Most of these sugars are added to foods and beverages during manufacturing." Provide some suggestions for lowering sugar intake that seem reasonable to you. (160)

Instead of:	Try:
Sweet desserts	
Soda or powdered drink mixes	
Sugar-coated cereals	
Candy	
Canned fruit in heavy syrup	
Sweet rolls or doughnuts	

2. Use Appendix A in your textbook or your NutriTrac software to predict the energy and carbohydrate content in the following one-day diet.

Foods	Kcal	Carbohydrate (grams)
Breakfast		
3/4 cup Cheerios cereal		
1 cup 2% milk		
1/2 cup orange juice		
Lunch		
3 ounces broiled hamburger		
1 hamburger bun		
1 ounce cheddar cheese		
1 tablespoon mustard		
1 cup 2% milk		
1 apple		
Dinner		
3 ounces broiled chicken		
1/3 cup rice		
1/2 cup broccoli		
1 teaspoon margarine		
TOTALS:	_____ kcal	_____ grams of carbohydrate

What percentage of kcal content does carbohydrate contribute to this diet? _________%

See page 62 of this Study Guide to check your numerical answers.

E. "Much lactose is lost when milk is made into cheese." Provide four tips to a person with lactose intolerance in both reducing symptoms and having a healthy diet. (148)

a.

b.

c.

d.

F. "Aspartame yields 4 kcal per gram but is about 200 times sweeter than sucrose." Briefly describe the current uses and controversies surrounding the use of the following alternative sweeteners. (165-166)

a. aspartame (NutraSweet)

b. saccharin

c. acesulfame-K (Sunette)

V. Applying nutrition to your life

"Although a desirable amount of sugar intake has not yet been set, less than 10%-15% of total energy intake is recommended." First pick a weekend or weekday that would reflect a day as your greatest consumption of sugar (sweet foods). Write down all the sugared (sweet) foods and beverages you ate for that day. Look up the number of teaspoons of sugar in these foods in Table 5-3. Record this information in the table below.

Sugars and sweet foods	Teaspoons of sugar

____________ total teaspoons

How many teaspoons of sugar did you eat?

Put an X on the scale below where your sugar consumption rates:

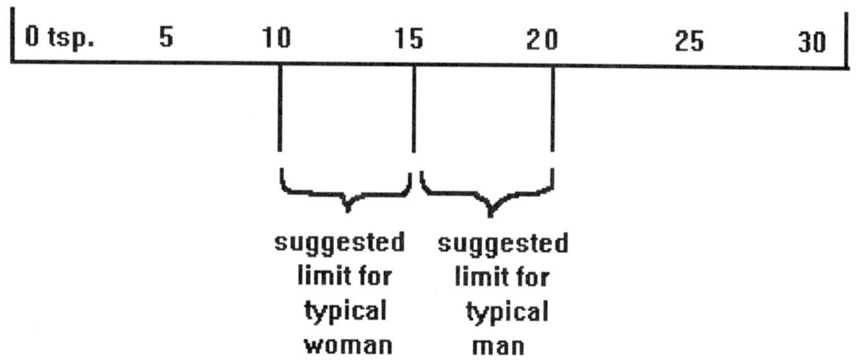

Did you exceed the limit suggested? How could you change your intake to reduce your sugar consumption?

VI. **Chapter 5 summary**

Fill in the blanks using the words listed at the end of this summary.

The monosaccharides in our diet include glucose, _________, and _________. Once absorbed by the small intestine and passed to the liver, these mostly leave as _________. The major disaccharides in nutrition are _________ (glucose plus fructose), _________ (glucose plus glucose), and _________ (glucose plus galactose). These are digested to form their _________.

Lactose is the sugar found in _________. _________ results when cells of the intestinal wall do not make sufficient _________, the enzyme necessary to digest lactose. Undigested lactose travels to the _________, resulting in symptoms such as abdominal gas, pain, and _______. Most people with lactose intolerance can tolerate cheeses, yogurt, and small amounts of milk, though tolerance to _________ as a whole is very individualistic.

Some _________ digestion occurs in the mouth. Carbohydrate digestion is finished in the _______. Some plant fibers are digested by the _________ present in the large intestine.

The major polysaccharides in our diet contain _________ glucose units linked together. _________ is an animal starch and acts as a storage form of carbohydrate in the liver.

The carbohydrates in our diet provide _________, protect against the needless metabolism of protein for energy, and provide _________ to foods. Many types of carbohydrates can be metabolized to __________ by bacteria on teeth. The acid can erode the tooth surfaces, leading to __________. The dietary fibers include _________, hemicelluloses, pectins, _________, mucilages, and lignins. Many of these provide mass to the ______, thus easing _________.

There is no _________ for carbohydrate. A minimal intake is 50 to 100 grams per day. About _________ of total energy intake is recommended. If inadequate carbohydrate intake continues for weeks at a time, the price is a loss of __________ protein, ketosis, and general weakness of the body. Diets high in _________ forms of carbohydrates are encouraged today to replace diets high in _________. Foods to emphasize are potatoes, grains, pastas, and vegetables.

Sugar intake should be limited to __________ of energy intake.

Diabetes is characterized by ________ blood glucose. Treatments for the disease can include a regulated carbohydrate/protein/fat consumption, use of insulin, weight loss, regular ________, and oral hypoglycemic agents, depending on the type of diabetes. True ________ is rare. ________ at every meal is part of the recommended therapy.

Use the following words to complete the summary:

acids
bacteria
body
cellulose
complex
dairy products
dental caries
diarrhea
energy
elimination
fat
flavor and sweetness
fructose
galactose
glucose
glycogen
gums
high
hypoglycemia
lactase
lactose
lactose intolerance
large intestine
maltose
milk
monosaccharides
multiple
physical activity
protein
RDA
small intestine
starch
stool
sucrose
10% to 15%
55%

Check your answers using the summary for Chapter 5 in your textbook; use the next page of this Study Guide for the last four answers.

Answers to selected questions

IV. D. 2. approximate kcalories = 80 + 120 + 60 + 225 + 160 + 100 + 0 + 120 + 60 + 165 + 80 + 25 + 45 = 1260 kcal

carbohydrate = 15 + 12 + 15 + 0 + 30 + 0 + 0 + 12 + 15 + 0 + 15 + 5 + 0 = 119 grams of carbohydrate

((119 x 4) / 1260) x 100 = 38% kcal as carbohydrates

VI. high; physical activity; hypoglycemia; protein

VII. Practice examination

Cover the answers on your initial attempt.

B 1. Cellulose, hemicelluloses, and lignins are fibers found in:

A. ripe fruits.
B. plant walls, skins, peels, and bran layers of grains.
C. pectin.
D. food additives such as guar gum.

C 2. In calculating the fiber content of your diet, the best value to use is the:

A. percentage of energy from carbohydrates.
B. total grams of carbohydrates.
C. dietary fiber value.
D. crude fiber value.

C 3. It is recommended that about ______ of your total energy intake come from carbohydrates.

A. 10%
B. 30%
C. 55%
D. 70%

A 4. Allen consumed 3200 kcal yesterday containing 100 grams of carbohydrate. What percentage of his energy intake came from the carbohydrates?

A. 12%
B. 25%
C. 50%
D. 75%

D 5. A high fiber diet:

A. is encouraged by a meat and potatoes menu.
B. is good insurance against diarrhea.
C. causes diverticulosis.
D. reduces transit time.

A 6. Which of the following is another name for glucose?

A. dextrose.
B. disaccharide.
C. fruit sugar.
D. all of the above.

C 7. The primary source of carbohydrates in the diet comes from which of the following group of foods?

A. milk and milk products.
B. breads, cereals, and grain products.
C. fruits and vegetables.
D. meat, fish, poultry, and beans.

B 8. The form of diabetes that often begins in late childhood and is characterized by the pancreas' inability to make insulin is called:

A. hypoglycemia.
B. insulin-dependent diabetes.
C. non-insulin-dependent diabetes.
D. hyperglycemia.

For questions 9 through 12 identify the following carbohydrates:

D	9.	animal starch	A. sucrose
B	10.	monosaccharide	B. glucose
C	11.	plant starch	C. amylose
A	12.	disaccharide	D. glycogen

B 13. Which of the following hormones lowers blood glucose?

A. glucagon.
B. insulin.
C. epinephrine.
D. cortisol.

D 14. The RDA for carbohydrates is:

A. 44 grams.
B. 800 RE
C. 50 to 55 milligrams.
D. nonexistent; there is no RDA for carbohydrates.

C 15. Aspartame:

A. is stable at high temperatures.
B. may cause cancer.
C. contains about 4 kcal per gram.
D. is a carbohydrate.

D 16. Polysaccharides are made of:

A. one molecule of sugar.
B. two monosaccharides linked together.
C. three monosaccharides linked together.
D. many monosaccharides linked together.

A 17. What is the major problem associated with a diet high in simple sugars?

A. lack of fiber
B. hyperglycemia
C. diabetes
D. dental caries

B 18. Dental caries is caused by:

A. sugar in the mouth eroding the tooth enamel.
B. acids produced by bacteria as they metabolize carbohydrates.
C. bacteria directly digesting tooth enamel.
D. saliva in the mouth.

B 19. When sucrose is digested it yields:

A. two maltose units.
B. glucose and fructose.
C. glucose and galactose.
D. fructose and galactose.

D 20. Sucrose is not as sweet as:

A. starch.
B. maltose.
C. galactose.
D. fructose.

B 21. To metabolize fats adequately, the diet should contain ______ grams of carbohydrates.

A. 20 to 25
B. 50 to 100
C. 100 to 200
D. 200 to 300

D 22. The best type of fiber to eat for reducing constipation is:

A. glycogen.
B. crude fiber.
C. soluble fiber.
D. insoluble fiber.

B 23. The chief function of carbohydrates we eat is to:

A. maintain body fat.
B. provide energy.
C. provide essential amino acids.
D. transport vitamin A.

C 24. A high-carbohydrate diet:

A. is necessarily fattening.
B. causes ketosis.
C. is protein-sparing.
D. forces glucose production from protein.

D 25. The symptoms of lactose intolerance are mainly caused by eventual lactose breakdown by bacteria in the:

A. mouth.
B. stomach.
C. small intestine.
D. large intestine (colon).

Chapter 6
Lipids

I. Points to consider

Chapter 6 is designed to allow you to:

1. List four classes of lipids and the role of each in nutritional health.
2. Differentiate between monoglycerides, diglycerides, and triglycerides.
3. Differentiate between saturated, monounsaturated, and polyunsaturated fatty acids in terms of structure and food sources.
4. Name the essential fatty acids and explain why they are called "essential."
5. Name the classes of lipoproteins and classify them according to their functions.
6. Discuss the implications of fat, including the omega-3 fatty acids, with respect to heart disease.
7. Identify hidden fat in foods and name available fat replacements.
8. Characterize the symptoms of heart disease and highlight some known risk factors.

II. Word parts

Complete the following exercise using words in Chapter 6.

Word part	Meaning	Examples
lip	lipid, fat	______________
phos	phosphorus	______________
philic	loving, affinity for	______________
phobic	fear	______________
tri	three	______________
hydro	water	______________

III. **Flash cards**

Cut out and review the flash cards for this chapter in Appendix A.

IV. **Review and synthesis**

A. 1. "Lipids are a diverse group of chemical compounds, but they share one main characteristic: they do not readily dissolve in water." Name three types of lipids, excluding fatty acids. (176)

a.

b.

c.

Briefly note the basic function of each.

The largest portion of fat in the food supply and in your body is in the form of____________________. (178)

A monoglyceride contains glycerol and how many fatty acids? _______ (178)

A saturated fatty acid contains how many C=C double bonds? _______ (176)

A polyunsaturated fatty acid contains how many C=C double bonds? _________ (177)

2. "The shorter chain length overrides the effect of saturation." The physical properties of a fat are determined by what two chemical characteristics? (177)

a.

b.

3. "The polyunsaturated fatty acids must become more saturated to solidify vegetable oils for use in shortenings and margarines." Name this process and briefly explain how it occurs. Then name two foods you eat that contain these types of fats. (189)

B. 1. "Alpha-linolenic acid is a major omega-3 fatty acid in foods; linoleic acid is the major omega-6 fatty acid." Provide one example to differentiate between the structures and the effects of products made from omega-3 and omega-6 fatty acids. (180)

2. The essential fatty acids are:

a.

b.

C. "When we store fats in adipose cells, we store little else."
Some functions of fat in the body are: (180-183)

a.

b.

c.

D. "Once the various dietary fats are digested and absorbed into the small intestine's cells, most of these are reformed into triglycerides." To review important concepts about lipid digestion, complete the following exercise. (186)

1. Fat digestion primarily occurs in the ___________.

2. Describe the role of bile in the digestion of fat.

3. Three end products of fat digestion are:

   a.

   b.

   c.

4. "Most of these fats are re-formed into triglycerides. These combine with phospholipids, protein, and cholesterol to form a __________________, one of many types of blood lipoproteins." The four major classes and functions of this and other lipoprotein compounds are: (186)

   a.

   b.

   c.

   d.

E. 1. "For foods in general, the highest nutrient density for fat is found in salad oil, butter, margarine, and mayonnaise; all contain about 100% of kcal as fat." (198) First rank the foods in fat content from 1 to 10, with 1 being the lowest in fat. Then use Appendix A in your textbook to determine how many grams of fat are actually in each of the foods below. Adjust serving size and therefore fat contribution so that all choices yield 250 kcal.

1)	croissant	______	6)	Snickers candy bar	______
2)	fried chicken	______	7)	cheddar cheese	______
3)	egg	______	8)	peanuts (oil roasted)	______
4)	roast beef (lean)	______	9)	green split pea soup	______
5)	white rice	______	10)	Triscuits (crackers)	______

Check your answers on page 76 of this Study Guide.

2. "Because many Americans are at risk for developing heart disease, the American Heart Association (AHA) promotes dietary changes aimed at reducing this risk." (193) Calculate the total kcal, grams of fat, and percentage of energy as fat in the following menu. Use Appendix A in your textbook or your NutriTrac software to assist you.

Foods	A kcal	B Fat (grams)
Breakfast		
1 cup whole milk		
1 egg (fried in 1 teaspoon margarine)		
2 ounces bacon		
2 slices white toast		
2 teaspoons margarine		
Lunch		
2 ounces peanut butter		
1/2 banana		
2 slices whole wheat bread		
1 cup whole milk		
Dinner		
4 ounces ribeye steak (no bone)		
2 tablespoons french dressing		
1/2 cup mixed salad		
1/2 cup grated cheese		
2 tablespoons sour cream		
1 baked potato		
1/2 cup green beans		
2 teaspoons margarine		
TOTAL	_____ kcal	_____ grams of fat

What percentage of energy intake does fat contribute to the previous diet?
_______________%

(HINT: [column B x 9] x 100/column A)

See page 74 of this Study Guide to check your numerical answers.

F. 1. "Heart disease is the major killer of Americans." What are three key controllable risk factors for heart disease? (208)

a.

b.

c.

2. Blood cholesterol may be raised by what specific components of the diet? Star the most significant component. (210-211)

a.

b.

3. Blood cholesterol may be lowered by what four specific diet changes?

a.

b.

c.

d.

See page 74 of this Study Guide to check your answers to parts 2 and 3.

G. "Currently five different types of fat replacements are available in the United States. Addition of these substances during manufacture yields products that to varying degrees satisfy consumers' desire for fat-reduced products that are still tasty." Name three fat replacements. Note how they are made and give an example of a current (or potential) food product each is found in. (202)

Name	How made	Example of food product
a.		
b.		
c.		

V. Applying nutrition to your life

How much fat and saturated fat does the AHA feel is too much for you? Determine this by doing some calculations.

First record the energy intake that is appropriate for you. Use the RDA for a rough guideline or the amount of kcal you ate listed on your diet analysis from Chapter 2.

kcal allowance ________________________

Now determine how many kcal from fat you could eat at this energy intake. Take 30% of the figure you wrote in the blank above.

kcal allowance x 0.30 = ____________ (kcal from fat)

Next, take this figure and divide it by the energy value for fat, 9 kcal/gram.

kcal from fat/9 = ________________ grams of fat

Finally, determine the most grams of saturated fat to be eaten. Take 10% of your kcal allowance, then divide the results by 9. This will give you the number of grams of saturated fat you should not exceed.

________________ grams of saturated fat

Consult your diet analysis in Chapter 2 in your textbook to see if your fat intake exceeds these values. If so, name three dietary changes you could make to stay within these guidelines.

a.

b.

c.

VI. Chapter 6 summary

Fill in the blanks using the words listed at the end of this summary.

Lipids are a group of relatively oxygen-poor compounds that do not readily dissolve in ________. Saturated fatty acids contain ________ C=C double bond(s); monounsaturated fatty acids contain ________ C=C double bond(s). If the C=C double bonds in the fatty acid begin at the third carbon atom from the methyl end ($-CH_3$), then the fatty acid is a(n) ___________ fatty acid. Fats composed of saturated fatty acids tend to be ______________ at room temperature; those with polyunsaturated fatty acids are usually _________ at room temperature. If the double bonds begin at the sixth carbon, it is a(n) __________ fatty acid. Both types of these fatty acids are essential parts of a diet. Cells use omega-3 fatty acids to synthesize hormone-like compounds that tend to reduce _________ and inflammatory responses in the body. Because many fish contain ample amounts of beneficial omega-3 fatty acids, eating fish about _________ a week is a good dietary practice.

Triglyceride is the major form of ________ in the body. Besides supplying essential fatty acids to the body, triglycerides supply _________, allow efficient energy storage, _________ and protect the body, transport fat-soluble vitamins, promote _________, and add flavor and texture to foods. Phospholipids are derivatives of triglycerides and form parts of _________; some act as _________. Cholesterol forms vital compounds for the body, such as hormones, parts of cell membranes, and _________. We eat cholesterol and _________ make it.

In the _________, pancreatic _________ digests triglycerides into small breakdown products. These are absorbed into _________ of the small intestine and mostly resynthesized into _________. These are incorporated into _________ and eventually enter the _________.

Fats are carried in the bloodstream by lipoproteins: chylomicrons, ___________, low density lipoproteins (LDL), and high density lipoproteins (HDL). Elevated _________ is associated with a high risk of heart disease, as is low _________.

_________ is the process of turning C=C double bonds in fatty acids into single bonds. Manufacturers hydrogenate fats to solidify vegetable oils for making shortenings and margarines and to reduce the breakdown of polyunsaturated fatty acids. This leads to less _________.

There is no RDA for fat. One needs about _________ of _________ daily to obtain the needed omega-6 _________. To lower a high blood cholesterol, one should mainly try to minimize the intake of _________ fatty acids. Major contributors of fat to our diet include animal foods, _________, and pastries. The fat substitute _________ will allow us to eat some snack products without consuming much fat.

Use the following words to complete the summary:

absorptive cells
bile
blood clotting
cells
cell membranes
chylomicrons
emulsifiers
energy
enzyme
essential fatty acids
fat
HDL
hydrogenation
insulate
LDL
liquid
lymphatic system
no
olestra
omega-3
omega-6
one
plant oils
rancidity
satiety
saturated
small intestine
solid
triglycerides
twice
very low density lipoproteins (VLDL)
water
whole milk
1 tablespoon

Check your answers using the summary for Chapter 6 in your textbook; use page 76 for the last three answers.

Answers to selected questions

IV. E. 1.

1. white rice - 0 grams of fat
2. green split pea soup - 5 grams
3. Triscuits - 9 grams
4. Snickers bar - 12 grams
5. croissant - 13 grams
6. fried chicken - 14 grams
7. roast beef - 15 grams
8. eggs - 18 grams
9. peanuts - 20 grams
10. cheddar cheese - 21 grams

E. 2.

kcal: 150 + 78 + 34 + 220 + 150 + 67 + 335 + 52 + 172 + 150 + 250 + 135 + 12 + 227 + 67 + 62 + 220 + 22 + 68 = 2465 kcal

fat: 8 + 5 + 4 + 19 + 2 + 8 + 28 + 0 + 3 + 8 + 13 + 13 + 0 + 19 + 8 + 6 + 0 + 0 + 8 = 152 grams

% energy from fat: (152 x 9)/2465 = 0.55 or 55%

F. 1. high blood pressure, smoking, high blood cholesterol

2. saturated fat*, cholesterol

3. eat less saturated fat, eat less cholesterol, eat less total fat, eat more soluble fiber

---

VII. Practice examination

Cover the answers on your initial attempt.

B 1. Which group of foods is highest in fat?

A. hamburger, french fries, and cupcake.
B. margarine, salad dressing, and corn oil.
C. cottage cheese, chicken, and soybeans.
D. eggs, cheese, and milk.
E. apple, spinach, and corn.

C 2. If an 1800-kcal diet contains 100 grams of fat, the percentage of kcal from the fat is:

A. 20 %.
B. 35 %.
C. 50 %.
D. 65 %.

A 3. The three-carbon "backbone" found in all triglycerides is called:

A. glycerol.
B. fatty acid.
C. acetic acid.
D. stearic acid.

C 4. Hydrogenation of fat does <u>NOT</u>:

A. increase shelf life.
B. make it harder.
C. make it more unsaturated.
D. reduce the tendency for oxidation.

D 5. Moderate fish consumption is primarily related to a decreased risk for heart disease because it lowers:

A. blood triglycerides.
B. blood cholesterol.
C. blood lipoproteins.
D. blood clotting activity.

B 6. If Jack Sprat truly could eat no fat, he would:

A. eliminate his risk for cancer.
B. not be able to make prostaglandins.
C. necessarily have a low serum cholesterol level.
D. have a high satiety value for his diet.

A 7. Cholesterol:

A. comes only from the animal food in our diet.
B. must be eaten in the diet.
C. is a breakdown product of lipids.
D. when present in the diet, is the leading cause of strokes.

C 8. The form of fat in food is primarily in the form of:

A. cholesterol.
B. fatty acids.
C. triglycerides.
D. phospholipids.

A 9. Which of the following is <u>NOT</u> an emulsifier?

A. glycerol.
B. bile acids.
C. lecithin.
D. diglycerides.

A 10. Emulsifiers and micelles are related in that:

A. an emulsifier forms a micelle.
B. a micelle produces an emulsifier.
C. both are classified as carbohydrates.
D. both operate primarily in the stomach.

A 11. Because lard is a solid at room temperature, most of its fatty acids are:

A. long and saturated.
B. short and saturated.
C. long and unsaturated.
D. short and unsaturated.

C 12. A symptom of an essential fatty acid deficiency is:

A. anemia.
B. hair color changes.
C. skin rash.
D. loss of hearing.

B 13. Bile acids are made from:

A. glucose.
B. cholesterol.
C. vitamin A.
D. prostaglandins.

B 14. The three major risk factors for heart disease do NOT include:

A. high blood cholesterol.
B. obesity.
C. hypertension.
D. smoking.

For questions 15 to 18, identify the following lipoproteins:

A. chylomicron
B. very low density lipoprotein
C. low density lipoprotein
D. high density lipoprotein

A 15. main carrier of dietary triglyceride in the bloodstream
C 16. linked to increase in heart disease risk
B 17. main carrier of triglyceride synthesized by the liver to body cells
D 18. linked to decrease in heart disease risk

For questions 19 to 22, indicate a concentrated food source for the following (use each food only once):

D 19. saturated fat
B 20. cholesterol
C 21. polyunsaturated fat
A 22. monounsaturated fat

A. canola oil
B. liver
C. safflower oil
D. butter

Match the following terms:

C 23. atherosclerosis
B 24. myocardial infarction
A 25. stroke

A. block in blood flow in brain
B. reduction in blood flow in the heart
C. buildup of fatty material in arteries

Answers to selected questions

VI. saturated; whole milk; olestra

Chapter 7
Proteins

I. Points to consider

Chapter 7 is designed to allow you to:

1. Describe how amino acids make up proteins.
2. Distinguish between essential (indispensable) and nonessential (dispensable) amino acids.
3. Explain why adequate amounts of each of the essential amino acids are required for protein synthesis.
4. List the primary functions of protein in the body.
5. When a healthy weight is given, calculate the RDA for protein for an adult.
6. Describe what is represented by positive nitrogen balance, negative nitrogen balance, and nitrogen equilibrium.
7. Distinguish between high-quality and low-quality protein and the sources of each, and describe how two low-quality proteins can be complimentary for each other and in turn provide all the essential amino acids.
8. Describe how protein energy malnutrition can eventually lead to disease in the body.

II. Word parts

Complete the following exercise using words in Chapter 7.

Word part	Meaning	Examples
amine	organic form of nitrogen	________
a	without	________
ost	bone	________
ov	egg	________

III. Flash cards

Cut out and review the flash cards for this chapter in Appendix A.

IV. Review and synthesis

A. 1. "Amino acids, the building blocks of proteins, contain a special form of nitrogen." The chemical elements (atoms) used to make amino acids are: (218)

a. c. e.

b. d.

2. "By linking various combinations of the 20 or so types of amino acids, the body synthesizes thousands of different proteins. Only correctly positioned amino acids can interact and fold properly to form the intended shape for the protein." Outline in your own words what is meant by this statement. Then within this context, define the term "denature." (223)

B. "We dismantle the proteins we get from foods and use the amino acids to assemble proteins we need." To review important concepts about protein digestion and absorption, imagine that for lunch you ate cheese pizza and drank a glass of 2% milk. Describe the digestion of the protein in the meal in each part of the digestive system. (224-225)

ORGAN	DIGESTIVE ACTIVITY
Mouth	
Stomach	
Small intestine	
Lumen (interior)	
Absorptive cells	

The final end products of protein digestion are:

After absorption, at which organ does the major end product first arrive?

C. "Therefore, proteins truly deserve their name, meaning 'to come first'." Describe four roles proteins serve in the body. (226)

a.

b.

c.

d.

D. 1. "Merely eating more protein does not guarantee a positive balance." Describe protein balance in practical terms. Then complete the following table. (230)

Positive protein balance is seen in:	Negative protein balance is seen in:	Protein equilibrium is seen in:

2. "Today the best estimate for the amount of protein required for nearly all adults is 0.8 grams of protein per kilogram of healthy body weight." Calculate your RDA for protein below. Healthy weights for heights are shown in Figure 10-6 in your textbook. Recall that 2.2 pounds equals 1 kilogram. (231)

E. "Vegetable proteins deserve more attention from Americans." Briefly justify this statement. (236)

F. "Both kwashiorkor and marasmus wreak havoc on infants and children." Account for these two effects of protein-energy malnutrition. Explain why deficiencies in energy and/or protein intake--as well as other factors--cause these effects. (236-239)

kwashiorkor

marasmus

V. Applying nutrition to your life

Use Appendix A in your textbook or the NutriTrac software to establish the energy and protein content of this one-day diet.

Food	kcal	Protein (grams)
Breakfast		
8 ounces orange juice		
1 egg		
2 slices white toast		
1 teaspoon margarine		
Lunch		
2 slices whole wheat bread		
2 teaspoons mayonnaise		
2 ounces cheddar cheese		
1 cup 2% milk		
1 medium apple		
Dinner		
4 ounces turkey roast		
1/2 cup green beans		
1 cup mashed potato		
2 teaspoons margarine		
Dessert		
6 graham crackers		
Totals	____kcal	____grams of protein

What percentage of kcal does protein contribute to the diet on page 80? ______%

Would this amount of food satisfy you in terms of:

1) protein needs?

2) energy needs?

3) typical daily intake?

Do you now think meeting protein needs is a weakness of your current diet?

See page 86 for answers to the calculations.

VI. Chapter 7 summary

Fill in the blanks using the words listed at the end of this summary.

_________ are the building blocks of proteins. Amino acids contain a very usable form of _________. Of the 20 or so types of amino acids found in food, nine _________ be consumed; the rest can be synthesized by the body.

High quality, also called "___________" protein foods contain ample amounts of all nine essential amino acids. Animal foods typically supply all of them in approximately the right amounts. _________, also called "incomplete" protein, lack sufficient _____ amino acids. This is typical of ________ foods, especially cereal grains.

Individual amino acids are ___________ together to form proteins. The sequential order of amino acids determines the protein's ultimate shape, and in turn ___________. If the three-dimensional shape of the protein eventually formed is unfolded -- ___________ -- by treatment with heat, acid or alkaline solutions, or other processes, the protein loses its biological activity.

Protein digestion begins in the _________, producing breakdown products called _________. In the small intestine, peptones eventually separate into ________. These travel via the _________ to the _________.

Important body components, such as muscles, __________, transport proteins, visual pigments, __________, some hormones, and immune factors are made up of proteins. The RDA for protein for adults is __________ grams per kilogram of healthy body weight. Typical American men consume about __________ grams of protein daily; __________ consume closer to 65 grams daily. Thus the American diet generally supplies plenty of __________.

Animal meats are the most nutrient-dense sources of protein. __________ contains over 80% of its energy content as protein. Plant foods generally contain less than __________ of their energy content as protein; however, __________ provide much protein when regularly part of a diet and contribute to a high-quality protein content for a meal if eaten with grain proteins or animal products. These sources are critical for __________ diets.

Undernutrition occasionally leads to __________ and marasmus. Kwashiorkor results primarily from an inadequate __________ and protein intake in combination with concurrent disease and infection. __________ results primarily from basic __________ -- a negligible intake of both protein and energy is seen.

Use the following words to complete the summary:

amino acids (2x)
complete
connective tissue
denatured
energy
enzymes
essential
function
kwashiorkor

legumes
linked
liver
low quality
marasmus
must
nitrogen
peptones
plant

portal vein
protein
starvation
stomach
vegetarian
water-packed tuna
women
0.8
20%
105

Check your answers using the summary for Chapter 7 in your textbook.

VII. Practice examination

Cover the answers on your initial attempt.

B 1. A buffer helps:

A. emulsify fats.
B. maintain a constant pH in a solution.
C. speed chemical reactions.
D. protect against plaque build-up in the arteries.

D 2. Which of the following is definitely not a protein?

A. antibody.
B. enzyme.
C. tendon.
D. glycogen.

A 3. Peptide bonds are formed:

A. by excluding water molecules.
B. by excluding hydrogen atoms.
C. by making emulsifiers.
D. when developing secondary structure.

B 4. Nonessential amino acids:

A. are not needed by the body.
B. are not needed in the diet.
C. are not needed daily, but weekly.
D. are found in only incomplete proteins.

B 5. The denaturing of protein:

A. destroys its amino acid order.
B. happens in the stomach.
C. increases its enzyme activity.
D. forms an emulsifier.

B 6. The order of amino acids in a specific protein determines its:

A. energy content.
B. function in the body.
C. biological value.
D. ability to form glucose.

D 7. Vegetarians who eat no animal products or nutrient-fortified products should supplement their diets with:

A. vitamin C.
B. magnesium.
C. vitamin A.
D. vitamin B-12.

B 8. Incomplete proteins:

A. do not follow the "all-or-none law."
B. are characteristic of plant foods.
C. are characteristic of animal foods.
D. are characteristic of snack foods.

C 9. The RDA for protein of a 60-kilogram (132-pound) woman is:

A. 36 grams.
B. 42 grams.
C. 48 grams.
D. 54 grams.
E. 60 grams.

D 10. Which is NOT true abcut kwashiorkor?

A. Protein needs are generally not met.
B. The child appears plump because of edema.
C. The child is at a high risk for infections.
D. The affected person is usually a very young infant.

A 11. In marasmus:

A. the child is often bottle-fed from birth.
B. protein needs are met.
C. muscle wasting is present, but it is hidden by edema.
D. preschool children, not infants, are typically affected.

A 12. Which of the following is NOT a protein?

A. maltose.
B. hemoglobin.
C. insulin.
D. collagen.

B 13. Which of the following does NOT provide mixtures of amino acids that are well balanced for humans?

A. corn and refried beans.
B. jello.
C. eggs.
D. macaroni and cheese.

B 14. A good protein intake recommendation is ______ of total energy intake.

A. 5% to 10%.
B. 10% to 15%.
C. 15% to 20%.
D. 20% to 25%.

B 15. Nutritional edema occurs when:

A. blood protein concentration is increased.
B. blood protein concentration is decreased.
C. the red cell number decreases.
D. there is a great change in blood hemoglobin concentration.

D 16. The food group that contributes no protein is:

A. milk, etc.
B. bread, etc.
C. vegetable.
D. fruit.

B 17. The chemical element (atom) found in all proteins, but not usually in fats or carbohydrates, is:

A. carbon.
B. nitrogen.
C. hydrogen.
D. oxygen.

D 18. An essential (indispensable) amino acid:

A. forms a complete protein.
B. is needed only by growing infants and children.
C. may prevent dermatitis.
D. cannot by synthesized by the body in sufficient amounts to meet the body's needs.

C 19. During pregnancy, nitrogen balance should be:

A. negative. B. in equilibrium. C. positive.

D 20. If a person takes in more protein than the body needs, the excess protein will be:

A. excreted in the urine.
B. converted to fat energy and stored in adipocytes.
C. used to provide energy for the body if needed.
D. B and C.

C 21. The RDA for protein is increased:

A. during mental stress.
B. after age 50.
C. during pregnancy and lactation.
D. whenever physical activity is increased.

A 22. One would expect to see a negative protein balance:

A. when certain hormones, such as thyroid hormone and cortisol, are released in excess amounts.
B. during pregnancy.
C. as one recovers from an illness.
D. in any healthy human being.

B 23. Proteins supply about 2% to 5% of the energy the body uses. It is not the primary source cells use because of:

A. the decreased amount of energy per gram available compared to carbohydrates.
B. the amount of metabolism and processing required by the liver and kidneys.
C. the inability of the body to make glucose from amino acids.
D. the complex planning required to obtain all nine essential amino acids in a typical diet.

C 24. Urea is synthesized from amino (NH) groups mostly in which tissue?

A. blood
B. kidneys
C. liver
D. small intestine

C 25. At which stage of life must a diet contain the highest percentage of protein as essential amino acids?

A. the very elderly
B. pregnant women
C. infants
D. young adults

Answers to selected chapter questions

V. kcal 110 + 78 + 185 + 34 + 170 + 66 + 230 + 120 + 82 + 160 + 22 + 220 + 68 + 180 = <u>1725</u>

protein 2 + 6 + 6 + 0 + 7 + 0 + 14 + 8 + 0 + 34 + 1 + 4 + 0 + 3 = <u>86</u>

percent energy from protein (86 x 4)/1725 = 0.199 or 20%

Chapter 8
Vitamins

I. Points to consider

Chapter 8 is designed to allow you to:

1. Define the term vitamin.
2. Classify the vitamins according to whether they are fat-soluble or water-soluble.
3. List the major functions and deficiency symptoms for each fat-soluble vitamin.
4. List the major functions and deficiency symptoms for each water-soluble vitamin.
5. List three important food sources for each fat-soluble vitamin.
6. List three important food sources for each water-soluble vitamin.
7. Describe toxicity symptoms from excess consumption of fat-soluble vitamins and certain water-soluble vitamins.
8. Distinguish between vitamins and nonvitamins, such as inositol and taurine.
9. Describe some cancer-causing mechanisms, and describe how diet and nutrition are related to their minimization.

II. Word parts

Complete the following exercise using words in Chapter 8.

Word part	Meaning	Example
xero	dry	________
osteo	bone	________
mal	poor	________
oid	like, resemble	________
malacia	softened	________
blast	immature cell	________
osis	condition of	________
cyte	cell	________

III. Flash cards

Cut out and review the flash cards for this chapter in Appendix A.

IV. Review and synthesis

A. "By definition, vitamins are essential organic (carbon-containing) substances needed in small amounts in the diet." Differentiate between the classes of vitamins using the terms in parentheses. Use one term twice if appropriate. (248-250)

	Fat-soluble	Water-soluble
Absorbed into (blood or lymph)		
Excess (easily excreted or poorly excreted)		
Excess (often toxic or not often toxic)		
Generally (form or do not form) coenzymes		
Generally (stable or unstable) during cooking		

B. "The water-soluble vitamins, particularly thiamin, vitamin C, and folate, can be destroyed with improper storage and excessive cooking." Provide suggestions for retaining the maximum amount of vitamins when storing, preparing, and cooking vegetables. (268)

1. Storing vegetables

   a.

   b.

2. Preparing and cooking vegetables

   a.

   b.

   c.

   d.

C. "For vitamin A, the current unit of measurement is the retinol equivalent (RE)." (256)

1. The provitamin forms of vitamin A are found in ____________________ foods,

   whereas the already active forms of vitamin A are found in ________________ foods.

2. The RDAs (from inside cover of your textbook) for men and women ages 19 to 50 years for vitamin A are:

   men ________________RE women ________________RE

D. "The net result of vitamin D hormone action is increased calcium and phosphorus deposition in bones." Describe how rickets could develop in childhood. (258)

E. "Functioning as a fat-soluble antioxidant, vitamin E resides mostly in cell membranes." (259)

1. How does vitamin E protect fats from breakdown?

2. What would be one health consequence if vitamin E was lacking in the diet?

3. How does the mineral selenium spare some of the body's need for vitamin E?

F. "Some of the vitamin K we absorb every day is synthesized by intestinal bacteria; most comes from our diets." (263)

1. List two groups of people who may develop vitamin K deficiency. Briefly explain your reasons for listing these groups.

   a.

   b.

2. Describe the most likely result from a vitamin K deficiency. Why would these symptoms appear?

G. "This shows how limited the body's stores of thiamin are and how important it is to consume thiamin-rich foods daily." Discuss two reasons, besides limited body storage of thiamin, why a two week alcohol binge could lead to a thiamin deficiency. (266)

H. "Taking a toxic dose is quite easy." Dispel the notion that high doses of all water-soluble vitamins are safe. (274)

I. "A key role of the folate coenzymes is helping to form DNA." What tissues are first affected by a folate deficiency? Why? (274)

J. "Vitamins yield no energy for the body." To review the fat-soluble vitamins and water-soluble vitamins, complete the following chart. (Use Tables 8-2 and 8-3 in your textbook to check your answers.)

	Major function(s)	Likely result of a long-term deficiency	Nutrient-dense food sources	Likelihood for toxicity and possible result(s)
Vitamin A				
Vitamin D				
Vitamin E				
Vitamin K				
Thiamin				
Niacin				
Riboflavin				
Pantothenic acid				
Biotin				
Vitamin B-6				
Folate				
Vitamin B-12				
Vitamin C				

V. Applying nutrition to your life

Do you really need a vitamin supplement?

Read the Nutrition Facts on five food items you eat tomorrow. If you eat breakfast cereal, make sure you include that food in your calculations. Also, include foods you feel are especially nutritious parts of your diet. Write down the percentage of the Daily Value for the following water-soluble vitamins. Then total the amounts for each vitamin.

Foods	1	2	3	4	5	Total % Daily Value
Vitamin A						______
Thiamin						______
Niacin						______
Riboflavin						______
Vitamin B-6						______
Folate						______
Vitamin C						______

Did you meet your needs as predicted by the Daily Value (100%) that day for all the vitamins listed?

Note: If there are large gaps between your intake and 100%, review the diet analysis you did for Chapter 2 in your textbook before deciding if a vitamin supplement is needed.

VI. Chapter 8 summary

Fill in the blanks using the words listed at the end of this summary.

Vitamins are compounds we need daily in small amounts from foods. They yield no energy themselves, but many contribute to energy-yielding chemical reactions in the body as well as promote growth and development. Many vitamins act as coenzymes, helping enzymes function. Vitamins A, D, E, and K are fat-soluble; the B vitamins and vitamin C are water-soluble.

Fat-soluble vitamins are absorbed along with dietary fat and are more poorly excreted from the body than are water-soluble vitamins.

Vitamin A consists of a family of compounds that includes several forms of ____________ vitamin A. ____________, such as beta-carotene, function as antioxidants and can also yield vitamin A. Vitamin A contributes to ____________, immune function, and cell development. Vitamin A is found in liver and fish oils; carotenoids are especially plentiful in dark green and ____________ vegetables. Vitamin A can be quite ____________, even when taken at just five times the RDA.

Vitamin D is both a ____________ and a vitamin. Human skin synthesizes it using sunshine and a cholesterol-like substance. If we don't spend enough time in the sun, foods such as fish oils and fortified ____________ can supply the vitamin. The active hormone form of vitamin D helps regulate blood calcium by influencing calcium absorption from the ____________. It also helps to regulate bone metabolism. Children who don't get enough vitamin D may develop ____________, and adults with inadequate amounts in the body develop ____________. Vitamin D is a very toxic substance. An intake just ____________ times the RDA can cause problems, especially in childhood.

Vitamin E functions primarily as an ____________. By donating electrons to electron-seeking free radical compounds, it neutralizes them. This effect shields cell membranes and red blood cells from ____________. Vitamin E is plentiful in ____________.

____________ helps blood clot. Some vitamin K absorbed each day comes from ____________ synthesis in the intestine, but most comes from foods, primarily ____________ vegetables. Vitamin K is poorly stored in the body, but our dietary intake alone is usually ____________.

Thiamin, ____________, and niacin play key roles as coenzymes in energy-yielding reactions. They help ____________ carbohydrates, fats, and proteins. ____________ and a poor diet can create deficiencies of these three nutrients. ____________ products are common sources of all three of these vitamins.

Pantothenic acid, which participates in many aspects of cell metabolism, is widely distributed among foods. Biotin, which participates in ___________ production, fat synthesis, and DNA synthesis, can be synthesized by bacteria in the intestine. In this fashion, we probably synthesize about ___________ our requirement for biotin. The rest comes from foods such as eggs and ___________.

Vitamin B-6 performs a vital role in protein metabolism, especially in synthesizing nonessential ___________. It also helps synthesize ___________ and performs other metabolic roles. Headaches, anemia, ___________, and vomiting result from a B-6 deficiency. Regular consumption of ___________ protein foods, cauliflower, and broccoli provides needed vitamin B-6. Taking high doses causes malfunction of the ___________ system.

Folate plays an important role in _________ synthesis. Symptoms of a deficiency are generally poor cell division in various areas of the body, anemia, ___________ inflammation, diarrhea, and poor growth. Good food sources are leafy vegetables, organ meats, and _________ juice. Great amounts of folate can be lost in cooking.

Vitamin B-12 is needed to metabolize folate and to maintain the ___________ surrounding nerves. A deficiency results in _________ (because of its relationship to folate) and nerve degeneration. ___________ people often absorb vitamin B-12 inefficiently. If so, they benefit from monthly injections of the vitamin. For others, a ___________ is unlikely because vitamin B-12 is highly concentrated in animal foods. Vitamin B-12 does not occur naturally in ___________ foods. ___________ need a supplemental source.

___________ is used mainly to synthesize collagen, a major protein for building connective tissue. A vitamin C deficiency results in ___________, which is evidenced by poor wound healing, pinpoint hemorrhages in the skin, and bleeding gums. Vitamin C also modestly enhances ___________ absorption. Fresh fruits and vegetables, especially __________ fruits, are generally good sources.

__________ is the second leading cause of death for adults in the United States; it affects different types of __________ and arises from many different causes. The process begins with an alteration in DNA, the __________ material in our cells. There are many ways to alter DNA, such as radiation from the sun, both natural and man-made chemicals, and the insertion of viral genes into human cells. Both _________ and physical inactivity are linked to increased risk for many types of cancer.

Use the following words to complete the summary:

alcoholism	five	orange
amino acids	genetic	osteomalacia
anemia	glucose	plant
animal	green, leafy	plant oils
antioxidant	half	preformed
bacterial	hormone	riboflavin
breakdown	insulation	rickets
cancer	intestine	scurvy
carotenoids	iron	sufficient
cells	metabolize	tongue
cheese	milk	toxic
citrus	nausea	vegans
coenzymes	nervous	vision
deficiency	neurotransmitters	vitamins
DNA	obesity	vitamin C
energy	older	vitamin K
enriched grain		water-soluble

Check your answers using the summary for Chapter 8 in your textbook; use the next page of this Study Guide for the last four answers.

Answers to selected questions

VI. cancer; cells; genetic; obesity

VII. Practice examination

Cover the answers on your initial attempt.

_C_ 1. The first symptom(s) of scurvy are:

A. dental caries.
B. depression and anxiety.
C. pinpoint hemorrhages under the skin.
D. pernicious anemia.

_B_ 2. Vitamin C is essential in the synthesis of a hydroxyproline residue found in:

A. ascorbic acid.
B. collagen.
C. leukocytes.
D. hemoglobin.

_B_ 3. Which of these meals lacks vitamin C?

A. corned beef, cabbage, fried potatoes, and milk
B. roast beef, carrots, noodles, and tea
C. spaghetti with tomato sauce, meatball, garlic bread, and diet soda
D. roast beef, broccoli, noodles, and coffee

_D_ 4. A deficiency of either of these two vitamins produces a similar type of anemia:

A. riboflavin and niacin.
B. thiamin and riboflavin.
C. pantothenic acid and biotin.
D. vitamin B-12 and folate.

_C_ 5. Choline is:

A. an enzyme.
B. part of bile.
C. part of lecithin.
D. a vitamin.

_C_ 6. Folate is found in small amounts in many foods, but the best sources are:

A. whole grain cereals.
B. cheese, eggs, and cream.
C. leafy, green vegetables and some fruits.
D. raw sugar, honey, and molasses.

C 7. The two foods high in vitamin B-6 are:

A. whole grains and vegetable oils.
B. citrus fruits and vegetable oils.
C. meat and dairy products.
D. orange fruits and vegetables.

B 8. Vitamin B-6 participates in:

A. iron absorption.
B. amino acid and protein metabolism.
C. release of energy from minerals.
D. utilization of calcium and phosphorus.

D 9. Alcohol interferes greatly with ________ absorption.

A. pantothenic acid
B. riboflavin
C. niacin
D. thiamin

D 10. The major sources of riboflavin in the American diet are:

A. whole grains.
B. green leafy vegetables.
C. citrus fruits and tomatoes.
D. dairy products.

C 11. A high intake of folate is dangerous because it:

A. means the person is eating too much protein.
B. is easily stored in the body.
C. can "mask" pernicious anemia.
D. causes neural tube defects

C 12. Thiamin is used for:

A. formation of polysaccharides.
B. formation of red blood cells.
C. energy release from nutrients.
D. collagen formation.

A 13. Each of the B vitamins functions as a(n):

A. part of a coenzyme.
B. electrolyte.
C. anticoagulant.
D. source of energy.

C 14. Pernicious anemia is primarily caused by a defect in:

A. vitamin B-12 intake.
B. vitamin B-12 excretion.
C. vitamin B-12 absorption.
D. vitamin B-12 interconversion.

D 15. Which vitamin participates in homocysteine metabolism?

A. vitamin B-12
B. folate
C. vitamin B-6
D. all of the above

D 16. Pantothenic acid is a part of the structure of:

A. pyruvate.
B. cobalamin.
C. glycogen.
D. coenzyme A.

D 17. Vitamins may be defined as:

A. inorganic compounds in food needed in small amounts for growth and maintenance of health.
B. organic compounds formed by the endocrine glands and necessary for growth and maintenance of health.
C. catalysts for hormones.
D. organic compounds in food needed in small amounts for growth and maintenance of health.

C 18. The only foods that generally provide ample amounts of vitamin C are:

A. meats.
B. milk and cheese.
C. vegetables and fruits.
D. breads and cereals.

C 19. Biotin is used for:

A. glucose absorption.
B. urea production.
C. fatty acid metabolism.
D. emulsification.

A 20. Which of the following statements is true for niacin?

A. It can be synthesized in the body from tryptophan.
B. It is an antioxidant.
C. It is water-soluble and therefore safe to administer in large doses.
D. It can be used to successfully cure anemia.

Match the vitamin to the appropriate deficiency disease.

C	21.	scurvy	A. riboflavin
D	22.	beriberi	B. niacin
F	23.	megaloblastic anemia	C. vitamin C
E	24.	pernicious anemia	D. thiamin
B	25.	pellagra	E. vitamin B-12
A	26.	cheilosis	F. folate
H	27.	vitamin A	G. red blood cell hemolysis
I	28.	vitamin D	H. xerophthalmia
G	29.	vitamin E	I. osteomalacia

B 30. Vitamin K is needed in the body for:

A. enzyme action.
B. blood clotting.
C. energy production.
D. strengthening bones and teeth.

D 31. Identify one function of vitamin D:

A. necessary for glucose metabolism.
B. prevents scurvy.
C. acts as an antioxidant.
D. aids in the absorption of calcium.

D 32. Which of the following substitutes for some of our need for vitamin E?

A. sodium
B. sulfur
C. silver
D. selenium

C 33. One of the last effects of vitamin A deficiency is:

A. anemia.
B. osteoporosis.
C. blindness.
D. hemorrhage.

D 34. The vitamin synthesized by bacteria in the intestine is:

A. E.
B. D.
C. A.
D. K.

A 35. Which of the following is <u>not</u> generally a true statement about fat-soluble vitamins?

A. Excess amounts are easily excreted from the body.
B. They can be consumed less frequently than the water-soluble vitamins.
C. They are bound to proteins when traveling in the blood.
D. They may accumulate to toxic amounts in the body.

D 36. Identify the best sources of beta-carotene:

A. whole grains, nuts, seeds, egg yolk, and plant oils.
B. lean meat, poultry, fish, and legumes.
C. corn, peas, beans, peaches, and asparagus.
D. pumpkin, carrots, squash, sweet potatoes, and apricots.

C 37. Which of the following symptoms would indicate a vitamin D deficiency in infants and young children?

A. abnormally high blood calcium
B. rupture of red blood cells
C. bowed legs
D. abnormally low blood calcium

D 38. Which of the following is <u>not</u> a good source of vitamin D?

A. sunshine
B. fatty fish
C. fortified milk and margarine
D. fruit, vegetables, and whole grains

__D__ 39. Vitamin K is found in:

A. seafood, iodized salt, and dairy products.
B. citrus fruits, cantaloupe, seeds, and nuts.
C. whole-grain cereals, milk, and cheese.
D. green, leafy vegetables and broccoli.

__B__ 40. Vitamin E functions in the body:

A. for maintenance of vision and health of skin, as well as growth of nails and bones.
B. as an antioxidant to prevent cell damage.
C. to calcify bones and teeth.
D. to supply energy and spare protein.

__C__ 41. The Council of Scientific Affairs of the American Medical Association recommends taking no more than ______ to ______ of the adult Daily Value for vitamins in supplement form.

A. 100% to 150%
B. 60% to 120%
C. 50% to 150%
D. 25% to 50%

__B__ 42. All adults should faithfully take a multivitamin at least once a day to prevent illness linked to deficiency in many nutrients.

A. True
B. False

Chapter 9
Water and Minerals

I. Points to consider

Chapter 9 is designed to allow you to:

1. Classify the minerals as major or trace minerals.
2. List conditions of the body, dietary factors, and other pertinent relationships that influence the absorption, retention, and availability of specific minerals.
3. List and briefly explain the functions of water in the body.
4. List key functions of the major and trace minerals.
5. Identify possible deficiency and toxicity symptoms associated with the major and trace minerals.
6. List at least two food sources for each of the major and trace minerals.
7. Describe the processes involving minerals that aid in maintaining bone health as well as those that aid in control of blood pressure.
8. Evaluate the use of mineral supplements with respect to their benefits and hazards to the body.

II. Word parts

Complete the following exercise using words in Chapter 9.

Word part	Meaning	Examples
penia	deficiency	________________
intra	inside	________________
extra	outside	________________
tens	to stretch	________________
myo	muscle	________________
hem	blood	________________
emia	in blood	________________
chrom	color	________________
goit	throat	________________

III. Flash cards

Cut out and review the flash cards for this chapter in Appendix A.

IV. Review and synthesis

A. "Depending on how much fat has been stored, an adult can survive for about 8 weeks without eating food but only a few days without drinking water." There are several sources of water, several routes of excretion, and many functions of water in the body. Sort the items in the box into the correct categories. (298)

Sources	Functions	Excretion
______	______	______
______	______	______
______	______	______
	______	______

1. evaporation
2. feces
3. solid food
4. beverages
5. acid-base balance
6. solvent
7. perspiration
8. temperature regulation
9. medium for transport
10. urine
11. metabolic water

B. "The ability to absorb minerals from a diet depends on many factors. The number listed in a food composition table for the amount of a mineral in a food is just a starting point for estimating the actual contribution the food will make to our mineral needs." Explain how moderation, balance, and variety in the diet promote optimum mineral absorption. (305)

C. "If we ate only unprocessed foods and added no salt, we would consume about 500 milligrams of sodium per day." (309)

1. Compare the sodium contents (per 100 kcal) of foods in the Food Guide Pyramid using Appendix A in your textbook.

Sodium (Na)
(milligrams per 100 kcal)

________	Milk (whole)
________	Cheese (cheddar)
	Vegetable
________	leafy (spinach)
________	other (corn)
________	Fruit (apple)
________	Breads and Cereals (enriched bread)
________	Meat (steak)
________	Egg
________	Fat (use margarine)

Note: 500 milligrams is the minimum requirement for health.

2. To what extent does sodium enter in the diet from natural foods versus manufactured foods based on this analysis?

D. "Bone strength depends on a person's bone mineral density. The more densely packed the bone crystals are, the stronger the bone structure." (344)

1. List 3 factors associated with bone maintenance versus bone loss.

Maintenance	Loss
a.	a.
b.	b.
c.	c.

2. Based on this information, what recommendations might you make to a 10-year-old girl to decrease her risk for osteoporosis in later years? (285)

E. "Minerals are vital to the functioning of many body processes." (288) List two major minerals that:

1. help maintain bone mass in the body

   a.

   b.

2. help maintain water balance in the body

   a.

   b.

3. help promote nerve function in the body

   a.

   b.

4. are necessary for the contraction and relaxation of the muscles

   a.

   b.

See page 112 of this Study Guide for possible answers.

5. Place a check mark when a food group makes an important contribution for a major mineral. Refer to Table 9-5 if you need help.

Food Group	Na	K	Cl	Ca	P	Mg
Milk and cheese						
Meat, fish, poultry, and beans						
Fruits and vegetables						
Breads and cereals						

F. 1. "Heme iron is absorbed more than twice as efficiently as the simple elemental iron called *nonheme iron*." List four factors that increase and four factors that decrease iron absorption. (326)

Increase	Decrease
a.	a.
b.	b.
c.	c.
d.	d.

2. "More Americans have an iron deficiency than iron-deficiency anemia, especially in America." Compare the effects of iron deficiency on the body to those resulting from iron-deficiency anemia. (327)

3. Provide four suggestions for increasing iron intake.

a.

b.

c.

d.

G. "Men drafted from the Pacific Northwest and the Great Lakes Region of the United States had a much higher rate of goiter than men from other areas of the country. The soils in these areas have very low iodide contents." (333)

1. One of the symptoms of iodide deficiency is an enlargement of the thyroid gland. Why does this gland enlarge as a result of this deficiency?

2. Briefly discuss the main reason iodide deficiency is now rare in the United States.

H. "Information about trace minerals is perhaps the most rapidly expanding area of knowledge in nutrition." Complete the following table. (339)

Trace mineral	Major function(s)	Likely result of long-term deficiency	Good food sources	Likelihood for toxicity and possible results
Zinc				
Copper				
Selenium				
Fluoride				
Chromium				

V. **Applying nutrition to your life**

"We consume about 1 liter (1 quart) of water a day in various liquids. Foods supply another liter of fluid; many fruits, vegetables, and beverages are more than 80% water. Water as a by-product of metabolism provides approximately 350 milliliters (1½ cups) of additional water." (301) Use your diet record from Chapter 1 in the textbook to examine your beverage intake in terms of amount and energy supplied (1 cup = 8 fluid ounces).

Beverage	Amount (cups) for the day	kcal
Water		-----------
Milk		
Fruit juices		
Soft drinks		
regular		
diet		
Coffee/tea		
Hot chocolate		
Sports drinks		
Alcoholic beverages		
TOTAL	__________ total cups	__________ total kcal
	__________ total milliliters (cups x 240)	

---

1. What was your primary beverage?

2. Were the energy-containing beverages generally nutritious beverages or non-nutritious beverages?

3. Did you meet the general guidelines of 1 milliliter of fluid per total kcal expended for the day? What one change do you think is needed in your beverage habits?

VI. Chapter 9 summary

Fill in the blanks using the words listed at the end of this summary.

Water constitutes ________ of the human body. Its unique chemical properties enable it to dissolve substances, as well as serve as a medium for chemical reactions, temperature regulation, and ___________. For adults, daily water needs are estimated at 1 milliliter per kcal _______. Many _______ are vital for sustaining life. For humans, animal products are the most bioavailable source of minerals. Supplements of minerals exceeding _____ of recommended amounts should be taken only under a physician's supervision because _______ and nutrient interactions are likely possibilities.

Sodium, the major positive ion found _______ cells, is vital in fluid balance and nerve impulse transmission. The American diet provides abundant ________ through processed foods and table salt. About 10% to 15% of the adult population is _________ for developing high blood pressure from consuming excessive sodium.

Potassium, the major positive ion found ________ cells, functions similarly to sodium. Milk, __________, and vegetables are good sources. ________ is the major negative ion found inside cells. It is important in digestion as part of gastric _________ and in immune function. Table salt supplies most of the chloride in our diets.

Calcium forms a vital part of bone structure and is also very important in ________, muscle contraction, nerve transmission, and cell metabolism. Calcium absorption is enhanced by stomach acid and the active ________ hormone. Dairy products are important calcium sources.

________ aids enzyme function and forms part of energy-containing molecules, cell membranes, and bone. It is efficiently absorbed and deficiencies are rare, although there is concern about the intake by _______ women. Good food sources are dairy products, bakery products, and meats. Sulfur is incorporated into certain vitamins and _________. Magnesium is a mineral found mostly in plants. It is important for _______ and heart function and as an activator for many enzymes. Whole grains (bran portion), vegetables, ______, seeds, milk, and meats are good food sources.

Iron absorption depends mainly on the form of iron present and the body's need for it. ________ iron from animal sources is better absorbed than the nonheme iron obtained primarily from plant sources. Consuming _________ simultaneously with iron modestly increases nonheme absorption. Iron operates mainly in synthesizing _________ and myoglobin and in the action of the immune system. Women are at great risk for developing iron deficiency, which decreases blood hemoglobin and red blood cell number. When this condition is severe enough to decrease the amount of oxygen carried in the blood, iron-deficiency _________ develops. Iron toxicity usually results from a genetic disorder called __________.

Zinc aids in the action of over 300 enzymes that are important for growth, development, immune function, __________, and taste. A zinc deficiency results in poor growth, loss of appetite, reduced sense of taste and smell, ______ loss, and a persistent rash. Zinc is best absorbed from animal sources. The most nutrient-dense sources of zinc are oysters, _______, crab, and beef. Good plant sources are whole grains, peanuts, and beans.

An important role of selenium is in decreasing action of _________ compounds. In this way, selenium acts along with vitamin E. Muscle pain, _________, and a form of heart disease may result from a selenium deficiency. Meats, eggs, fish, and shellfish are good animal sources of selenium. Good plant sources include grains and seeds. Iodide forms part of the ______ hormones. A lack of dietary iodide results in the development of an enlarged thyroid gland or __________. Iodized salt is a good food source. Fluoride incorporated into teeth during development makes them resistant to _________. Most Americans receive the bulk of their fluoride from fluoridated _______ and toothpaste.

Copper is important for ______metabolism, collagen cross-bonding, and other functions. A ________ deficiency can result in an iron-deficiency type anemia. Copper is found mainly in some seafoods, legumes, and ________.

Chromium aids in the action of _______. Egg yolks and whole grains are good sources of chromium. Manganese and __________ are used by various enzymes. Human needs for other trace minerals are so low that deficiencies are uncommon.

Blood pressure is expressed by two numbers. The higher number represents __________ blood pressure, the pressure in the arteries when the heart actively pumps blood. The second value is for __________ pressure, the arterial pressure when the heart is relaxed. __________ is usually defined as systolic pressure exceeding ________ mm Hg or diastolic blood pressure exceeding 90 mm Hg. A variety of factors affecting blood pressure include age, atherosclerosis, __________, race, and sodium and _______ intake.

Bone loss and ________ is linked to low calcium intake. Women are particularly at risk for this condition and should get plenty of calcium and _______. _______ replacement at menopause is currently the most accepted way to stop significant adult bone loss in women after menopause.

Use the following words to complete the summary:

alcohol	fruits	lubrication	sodium
amino acids	goiter	minerals	systolic
anemia	hair	molybdenum	thyroid
at risk	heme	muscle wasting	toxicity
blood clotting	hemochromatosis	nerve	vitamin C
chloride	hemoglobin	nuts	vitamin D
copper	high blood pressure	obesity	water
dental caries	hydrochloric acid	osteoporosis	whole grains
diastolic	inside	outside	wound healing
elderly	insulin	phosphorus	50% to 70%
estrogen	iron	physical activity	140
expended		shrimp	150%
free radical			

Check your answers using the summary for Chapter 9 in your textbook; use the next page of this <u>Study Guide</u> for the last nine answers.

Answers to selected questions

IV. E. 1.a. calcium, b. phosphorus; 2.a. sodium, b. potassium; 3.a. chloride, b. sodium; 4.a. magnesium, b. calcium

VI. systolic; diastolic; hypertension; 140; obesity; alcohol; osteoporosis; physical activity; estrogen

VII. Practice examination

Cover the answers on your initial attempt.

Match the letter to the appropriate mineral.

Answer	No.	Mineral	Letter	Description
H	1.	cobalt	A.	aids transport of oxygen
B	2.	copper	B.	aids in iron metabolism
D	3.	chromium	C.	associated with control of metabolic rate
C	4.	iodide	D.	contributes to normal metabolism of blood glucose
A	5.	iron	E.	needed for wound healing
F	6.	manganese	F.	needed for activity of enzymes used in carbohydrate metabolism
G	7.	selenium	G.	works with vitamin E
E	8.	zinc	H.	part of vitamin B-12
I	9.	fluoride	I.	strengthens tooth crystal

D 10. Iron is rapidly depleted from the body during:

A. vigorous exercise.
B. high calcium absorption.
C. rapid weight loss.
D. blood loss.

A 11. The most reliable food sources of zinc is (are):

A. meats and seafood.
B. orange juice.
C. dark green vegetables.
D. iodized salt.

B 12. Iron absorption from plant sources can be increased by ______ in the meal.

A. phytic acid
B. vitamin C
C. phosphates
D. fiber

A 13. Which of the following does not have antioxidant properties?

A. zinc
B. vitamin C
C. vitamin E
D. selenium

A 14. If an adult male is anemic, the first cause a physician suspects is:

A. blood loss.
B. cirrhosis of the liver.
C. a poor diet.
D. kidney disease.

D 15. Iodide deficiency results in:

A. anemia.
B. scurvy.
C. osteomalacia.
D. goiter.

B 16. High intakes of iron in certain people can lead to:

A. anemia.
B. liver damage.
C. hypertension.
D. ulcers.

D 17. Calcium is used in the body for:

A. enzyme regulation in cells.
B. excitability of nerves and muscles.
C. blood coagulation.
D. all of the above.

B 18. About how much fluid does the average adult take in as fluid and then excrete as urine per day?

A. 1 cup B. 4 cups C. 10 cups D. 20 cups

A 19. Calcium absorption is aided by:

A. vitamin D.
B. phosphorus and fiber.
C. oxalate and phytate.
D. all of the above.

A 20. The mineral that is part of the green pigment, chlorophyll, is:

A. magnesium. B. calcium. C. iron. D. selenium.

B 21. If enough calcium is not consumed:

A. heart rate will slow.
B. calcium will be removed from bone.
C. nerve impulses will cease.
D. caries will occur in the teeth.

A 22. Which of the following is not a function of water in the body?

A. acts as an antioxidant
B. allows for the excretion of wastes
C. allows for transport of many nutrients
D. helps dissolve certain substances

D 23. The sodium content of the diet of most Americans is ______ the amount needed in the body.

A. slightly in excess of
B. only a small percentage of
C. equal to
D. much in excess of

A 24. Which of the following factors below does not explain the high incidence of osteoporosis in postmenopausal women?

A. Women have higher intakes of calcium than men.
B. Women are living longer today.
C. Weight reduction diets are common among women.
D. Fall in estrogen status after menopause leads to bone loss.

D 25. The mineral found in highest concentration in intracellular fluid (inside the cell) is:

A. sodium. B. chloride. C. chromium. D. potassium.

C 26. Edema represents:

A. fluid loss from dehydration.
B. too much base in body fluids.
C. fluid in the extracellular space.
D. too much acid in body fluids.

D 27. Which of the following is the best food source of calcium?

A. tomato juice B. butter C. spinach D. yogurt

D 28. Significant food sources of potassium do <u>not</u> include:

A. orange juice. B. dried fruits. C. bananas. D. cheese.

C 29. Most water is lost daily via:

A. the skin. B. the lungs. C. urine. D. feces.

B 30. Most of the dietary phosphorus for Americans comes from:

A. fruits and vegetables.
B. dairy products and meat.
C. whole grains.
D. sugar and fat.

B 31. In a comfortable environment, water needs are about:

A. 1 milliliter per pound of weight.
B. 1 milliliter per kcalorie expended.
C. 1 milliliter per square centimeter of body surface area.
D. 1 milliliter per kilogram of body weight.

B 32. Magnesium functions:

A. in prevention of edema.
B. as a cofactor in energy metabolism.
C. as part of the thyroid hormone.
D. in the transport of oxygen.

D 33. Chloride:

A. is the body's principal intracellular electrolyte.
B. is necessary for protein synthesis in cells.
C. protects bone structure against decalcification.
D. helps maintain gastric acidity.

B 34. Almost all (99%) of the calcium in the body is used to:

A. maintain blood clotting.
B. strengthen bones and teeth.
C. provide energy for cells.
D. regulate the transmission of nerve impulses.

B 35. The calcium RDA for an adult over age 24 can essentially be met by consuming as part of an otherwise varied diet:

A. 1 cup of spinach.
B. 2 cups of milk.
C. 1 quart of milk.
D. a variety of plant foods.

Chapter 10
Weight Control

I. Points to consider

Chapter 10 is designed to allow you to:

1. Describe the uses of energy by the body and what constitutes energy balance.
2. Outline physiological and environmental factors that influence food intake.
3. Describe various ways of categorizing obesity.
4. Outline the risks to health posed by obesity.
5. List and discuss factors affecting energy balance in obesity with respect to nature and nurture.
6. Describe why and how reduced energy intake, behavior modification, and increased physical activity fit into a weight loss plan.
7. Outline the benefits and hazards of various weight-loss methods for severe (morbid) obesity.
8. Evaluate fad weight reduction diets and determine which are unsafe, doomed to fail, or both.

II. Word parts

Complete the following exercise using words in Chapter 10.

Word part	Meaning	Examples
horm	impulse	________________
mes	middle	________________
morph	form, shape	________________
ba	stand	________________
therm	heat	________________
calor	heat	________________
plas	mold, shape	________________
morbid	characterized by disease	________________

III. **Flash cards**

Cut out and review the flash cards for this chapter in Appendix A.

IV. **Review and synthesis**

A. "How much food energy is contained in a meal? A bomb calorimeter is used to determine the amount of energy in a food." Describe how a bomb calorimeter works. (354)

B. "The amount of energy used for basal metabolism depends primarily on lean body mass." Below are listed additional influences on basal metabolism. Explain briefly how each factor helps determine the metabolic rate (HINT: Does it increase it, decrease it, etc?). (355)

a. amount of body surface

b. gender

c. body temperature

d. thyroid hormone levels

e. age

f. nutritional state

g. pregnancy

C. "A predictable relationship exists between the body's use of energy and oxygen." Name and contrast the two methods of measuring energy use by the body. (358)

a.

b.

D. 1. "The next time you pick up a candy bar or ask for second helpings, remember the physiological and psychological influences on eating behavior. Body cells (brain, stomach, intestine, liver, and other organs), hormones (like cortisol), and social customs all influence food intake." Under each factor list two specific structures or mechanisms that influence us to begin eating or to end the process.

	Hunger	Appetite
Begin eating	a.	a.
	b.	b.
Stop eating	a.	a.
	b.	b.

2. "Almost everyone has encountered a mouthwatering dessert and devoured it, even on a full stomach." What drives your feeding behavior? List 3 possible factors and rank them according to the relative importance you think they have. (360)

a.

b.

c.

E. "We focus on body weight-for-height standards in clinical settings mainly because these are easier to measure than total body fat." Discuss two approaches to the definition of healthy body weight. (363)

a.

b.

F. 1. "Health risks associated with obesity actually apply only to people who are overfat." For the following health problems associated with excess body fat, list a possible reason why obesity can cause this health problem. (366)

Health problem	Partially attributed to
Adult-onset diabetes (NIDDM)	
Pulmonary disease	
Hypertension (high blood pressure)	
Coronary heart disease	
Bone and joint disorders	
Gallbladder stones	
Various cancers	

2. "More than half of body fat lies directly under the skin." Describe two ways the amount of body fat can be estimated. (366)

a.

b.

3. "Body weight is actually a crude measure of obesity." Briefly describe three methods used to diagnose the extent of obesity. These also predict the degree of associated health risks. (367)

Degree of confidence	Method	Cutoff value
Rough estimate	a.	
	b.	
Sensitive estimate	c.	

G. 1. "We also inherit specific body types, such as pencil-thin or muscular." List three factors that tend to increase the risk of obesity. Classify each as primarily "nature" or "nurture". (370-371)

a.

b.

c.

2. State three reasons why adult-onset obesity could possibly develop in your adult years.

a.

b.

c.

H. "They can be nurtured into gaining weight, allowing their natural tendency for obesity to blossom." Complete this table for a hamburger sandwich, a regular serving of french fries, and a strawberry milkshake. Recall the "4-9-4" relationship. Do the totals surprise you?

	Carbohydrate (grams)	Fat (grams)	Protein (grams)	Kcal
Quarter Pounder	29	24	25	________
French fries	26	12	3	________
Milk shake	62	9	9	________
Totals:	______	______	______	________

I. 1. "The plan should contain common foods. There is no magical food that can speed weight loss." What three components provide the best approach to weight reduction? (378)

a.

b.

c.

2. List the two criteria that indicate weight loss has been successful.

   a.

   b.

J. "New habits often need to replace defeating ones. For example, limiting eating to a single room in the house might eliminate television snacking." List some techniques that help apply behavioral principles to a weight-loss plan. (385)

   1. Stimulus control

      a. Shopping

      b. Plans

      c. Activities

      d. Holidays and parties

   2. Eating behavior

   3. Reward

   4. Self-monitoring

   5. Cognitive restructuring

K. "The easiest way to increase physical activity is to make it part of a daily routine." What are three benefits of increased physical activity in a weight-loss program? (383)

a.

b.

c.

L. "Underweight people should replace such foods as diet soft drinks with good energy sources like fruit juices." List three practices a person could follow to gain weight. (390)

a.

b.

c.

M. "The source of carbons for this glucose is mostly protein tissue." Describe why initial weight loss can be so rapid on a low-carbohydrate diet. (398)

V. Applying nutrition to your life

Choose a "diet" advertisement or article from a newspaper or magazine.

1. List two statements in the article that force you to question the worth of the plan.

   a.

   b.

2. Does your article cite an authority? If so, whom?

3. What credentials are given for this authority?

4. Overall, is the information in your article reliable? To what extent is it based on testimonials or unsubstantiated claims?

5. Consider these potential characteristics for the diet advice. Answer yes or no in the space provided.

   a. Is it nutritionally balanced? ______

   b. Will energy intake actually be reduced? ______

   c. Does it provide for a variety of typical foods? ______

   d. Is it economical? ______

   e. Will it teach new eating habits? ______

   f. Can it be followed with modifications after weight is lost? ______

6. Note any hazards or ill effects that might result from this particular diet.

VI. Chapter 10 summary

Fill in the blanks using the words listed at the end of this summary.

Energy ________ is energy intake minus energy output. __________ energy balance occurs when energy output surpasses energy intake, resulting in weight _______. _______ energy balance occurs when energy intake is greater than energy output. The result is weight ______.

Groups of cells in the hypothalamus and other regions in the _______ affect ________, the primarily internal desire to find and eat food. These cells may monitor nutrients and other substances in the ______ and read low amounts as a signal to promote feeding.

A variety of external (appetite-related) forces affect ______. Hunger cues combine with appetite cues, such as easy availability of food, to promote feeding. In America the major determinants of food intake are probably ______-driven forces because food is so readily available. The more _________ influences affecting food consumption are often suppressed or ignored.

Basal metabolism, the thermic effect of food, and _________ account for most of the body's energy use. _________, the minimum energy needed to keep the resting body alive, is primarily determined by _________, amount of body surface, and thyroid hormone. The _________ of food is energy the body uses to digest, absorb, and process nutrients recently consumed.

The body's energy use can be measured directly from ________ or indirectly from _______. Formulas based on various combinations of body weight, height, and age estimate the body's energy needs.

A person of ______ weight shows good health and performs daily activities without weight-related problems. A ________ (weight [in kilograms] ÷ height^2 [in meters]) of _______ is one measure of healthy weight, although weight in excess of this value may not lead to ill health. This suggests that healthy weight is best determined in conjunction with a thorough _______________ by a ________.

Obesity can be defined along several dimensions:

1. a total body fat exceeding _________ in men and 30% to 35% in women

2. a body mass index value over about ______

3. weighing ______ more than healthy body weight

Fat distribution predicts health risks from obesity. ________ body fat storage (characterized by a large abdomen and small buttocks and thighs) means higher risks of high blood pressure, heart disease, and diabetes than with lower body obesity (small abdomen and larger buttocks and thighs).

________ factors influence basal metabolism and body shape, and so influence the tendency to obesity. How one is raised (or nurtured) also influences obesity, because _________ often develop similar eating habits and activity patterns. Obesity may essentially be nurture allowing nature to be expressed.

When considering a treatment for obesity, remember: (1) a focus on healthy ______ rather than weight loss per se is more appropriate for many potential and current dieters; (2) the body ________ weight loss; (3) because obesity is difficult to reverse, the goal is ________; (4) lose weight mostly from _________, not mostly from muscle and other lean tissues; and (5) ________ weight loss and quick regain can be harmful to physical and ______ health.

A ________ weight-loss diet should meet a dieter's nutritional needs by following the Food Guide Pyramid. A good plan should adapt to the person's ________, encourage readily obtainable foods, strive to change poor eating habits, and promote regular _________ activity. It should also insist that the dieter see a physician if weight is to be lost ________ or if the person is over 35 years of age and plans to perform substantially greater physical activity than usual.

A pound of adipose fat tissue--gained or lost--represents approximately ________ kcal. If energy output ________ energy intake by about 400 kcal per day, one can lose a pound of fat storage per a week. We can best cut calories by decreasing intake of ________ foods.

Increasing physical activity sheds pounds. A good goal is to expend an extra ________ kcal or more in vigorous activity each day. ________ helps weight-loss programs because present habits may encourage overeating and discourage weight maintenance. Specific behavior modification techniques, such as _________ and self-monitoring, help change problem behaviors.

Severe obesity may require (1) gastric ________ to reduce stomach volume to approximately 50 milliliters, or (2) very low calorie diets, containing 400 to 800 kcal per day. Only people who _______ at more conservative approaches to weight loss should use these procedures.

______ can be caused by a variety of factors, such as excessive physical activity and genetic background. Sometimes being underweight requires _____ intervention. A physician should be consulted first to rule out ongoing _____. The underweight person may need to increase ______ and learn to like new ________ foods. In addition, encouraging a regular meal and snack _______ aids in weight gain and maintenance. A physically active person can reduce aerobic activity and substitute some _____________.

Over-the-counter weight-loss medications include ________, other mild stimulants, and fiber pills. None of these, however, replace a good diet, behavior changes, and physical activity.

_________ probably make more unreasonable, unproven, and dangerous claims for weight _____________ treatments than for any other person. So-called _____________ show up everywhere -- television, _____________, and newspapers. The ancient advice still applies: "Let the buyer ______________." Some common characteristics of _________ diets are (1) they promote ______________ weight loss but little ___________ loss takes place, and (2) they limit food ___________ and dictate specific ________.

Use the following words to complete the summary:

appetite	health evaluation	quick
balance	healthy	rapid
basal metabolism	heat output	rapidly
behavior modification	high fat	resists
beware	hunger	rituals
blood	lean body mass	satiety
body mass index	lifestyle	schedule
brain	loss	selections
cures	magazines	sound
diet quacks	medical	stimulus control
disease	negative	surgery
emotional	obesity	thermic effect
energy-dense	oxygen uptake	underweight
exceeds	phenylpropanolamine	upper
fad	physical	weight training
fail	physical activity	19 to 25
family members	physician	20%
fat	physiological	25%
fat storage	portion size	27 to 30
gain	positive	200
genetic	prevention	2700
habits		

Check your answers using the summary for Chapter 10 in your textbook; use page 130 of this Study Guide for the last eleven answers.

VII. Practice examination

Cover the answers for your initial attempt.

_B_ 1. Decreasing energy intake by about 400 kcal per day would mean a loss of about one pound of body fat stores in:

A. 2 days.
B. 7 days.
C. 10 days.
D. 14 days.

_C_ 2. If remaining at rest, an adult would use about how many kilocalories in a day?

A. 500 B. 800 C. 1400 D. 2500

D 3. Thermic effect of food represents the energy cost of:

A. chewing food.
B. peristalsis.
C. basal metabolism.
D. digesting, absorbing, and packaging nutrients.

C 4. A significant health hazard from obesity is:

A. ulcers.
B. diverticulosis.
C. diabetes.
D. emphysema.

For questions 5 to 12 indicate the effect of each of the following conditions on basal metabolism. (You may use A, B, and C more than once.)

A. increases it B. decreases it C. has no effect

A 5. more lean body mass
A 6. fever
B 7. fasting
A 8. pregnancy
A 9. large body surface area
C 10. mental thought
B 11. weight loss diet
B 12. aging

C 13. The hypothalamus:

A. increases metabolism for more efficient use of energy.
B. drives the psychological need for hunger.
C. contains a regulatory feeding center.
D. stops working after age 65.

C 14. A hormone involved in regulating basal metabolism is:

A. insulin.
B. gastrin.
C. thyroid hormone.
D. glucagon.

B 15. What percentage of a day's total energy need is used for digesting, absorbing, transporting, and storing nutrients?

A. 1% to 3%
B. 5% to 10%
C. 15% to 20%
D. 25% to 30%

C 16. What body fat concentration is the cutoff for obesity in men?

A. 10% B. 15% C. 25% D. 30%

D 17. An example of a behavior modification technique for weight control is:

A. always clean your plate when you eat.
B. have someone criticize you if you overeat.
C. feel guilty after you overeat.
D. keep a record of your eating habits so you can see what situations cause you to overeat.

D 18. Probably the most important reason for obesity today in the United States is:

A. set-point problems.
B. genetic selection.
C. "eating on the run".
D. inactivity.

D 19. Problems encountered with the use of drugs to lose weight include:

A. drugs may produce serious side effects.
B. many drugs induce the loss of body fluid but not body fat.
C. drugs do not lead to permanent changes in eating habits.
D. all of the above.

B 20. A general weight reduction diet should contain no less than:

A. 600 to 800 kcal per day.
B. 1000 to 1200 kcal per day.
C. 1500 to 1800 kcal per day.
D. 2000 to 2200 kcal per day.

A 21. People on weight reduction diets should minimize choices from:

A. high-fat foods.
B. breads and rolls.
C. potatoes.
D. meat.

D 22. A weight reduction program can be considered successful only when the weight loss:

A. is done without harming one's health.
B. is maintained permanently.
C. includes loss of body fat, body protein, and body water.
D. A and B

A 23. The best approach for weight loss is to:

A. reduce daily energy intake and increase energy expenditure.
B. avoid foods containing carbohydrates.
C. greatly increase protein intake to prevent body protein loss.
D. cut down on water intake.

C 24. What is usually the major factor that explains variability in the energy needs of two healthy men of similar age and size?

A. brown adipose tissue metabolism
B. basal metabolism
C. physical activity
D. type of diet consumed

C 25. Which of the following foods often is high in fat?

A. 1% milk
B. bread
C. meat
D. green vegetables
E. fruits

B 26. A reasonable weight-loss goal is:

A. no more than 1/4 pound per week.
B. 1 to 2 pounds per week.
C. 5 to 6 pounds per week.
D. depends on one's dominant gland.

D 27. A low-carbohydrate diet causes:

A. an increase in extracellular fluid.
B. glycogen synthesis.
C. increased rate of normal metabolism.
D. use of muscle tissue to produce glucose.

A 28. The most effective treatment for obesity is:

A. an energy intake less than energy output.
B. diuretic therapy.
C. use of hormones to increase basal metabolism.
D. a high-protein diet.

B 29. A major weakness of a very low-fat diet is:

A. essential fatty acid deficiency.
B. relative lack of satiety.
C. too little fiber.
D. too much linoleic acid.

C 30. When using physical activity to help lose weight, the key is:

A. intensity.
B. improving sports skills.
C. duration and regularity.
D. doing it at 6 AM.

A 31. Initial weight loss on a fad diet is often:

A. water, glycogen, and lean tissue.
B. abdominal fat.
C. sex-specific fat.
D. edema.

B 32. Behavior modification in obesity treatment includes:

A. following the physician's orders to the letter.
B. understanding and correcting poor dietary habits.
C. very low calorie diets.
D. gastric bypass surgery.

A 33. The intent of gastroplasty (stomach stapling) is to:

A. limit stomach volume.
B. speed transit time.
C. limit ability for absorption.
D. prevent snacking.

Answers to selected questions

VI. phenylpropanolamine; diet quacks; loss; cures; magazines; beware; fad; quick; fat; selections; rituals

---

Chapter 11
Nutrition: Athletics and Fitness

I. Points to consider

Chapter 11 is designed to allow you to:

1. Identify how regular physical activity can have a beneficial effect on the body.
2. Define metabolism and explain what is meant by anabolic and catabolic pathways.
3. Identify the major sources of energy for the body and illustrate various ways cells obtain ATP energy.
4. Show an understanding of glycolysis, differentiating between its aerobic and anaerobic aspects.
5. Describe the various energy systems used by muscles and when each is used by the muscle.
6. Examine the importance of carbohydrate in an athlete's diet and the importance of carbohydrate intake to athletic training.
7. Show an understanding of the importance of maintaining stores of various vitamins and minerals during athletic training.
8. Outline the importance of water, sports drinks, or both during physical activity.
9. Define ergogenic aids and describe their effects on an athlete's performance.

II. Word parts

Complete the following exercise using words in Chapter 11.

Word part	Meaning	Examples
metabo	change	______________
anabo	to build up	______________
catabo	breakdown	______________
tri	three	______________
di	two	______________
post	after	______________
glyco	sugar	______________

III. Flash cards

Cut out and review the flash cards for this chapter in Appendix A.

IV. Review and synthesis

A. 1. "Essentially, adenosine triphosphate (ATP) is the immediate source of energy for body functions." Briefly define ATP and describe the process of how ATP is formed. (409)

2. "Carbohydrates are an important fuel for muscles. The most useful form of carbohydrate fuel is the simple sugar glucose." Describe the basic process of glycolysis and explain the difference between its two pathways--aerobic and anaerobic. (410)

B. "The main advantages of PCr is that it can be activated instantly and can replenish ATP at rates fast enough to meet the energy demands of the fastest and most powerful actions, including jumping, lifting, throwing, and sprinting." Table 11-3 describes several energy systems used by muscle cells. Complete the following table, indicating when various energy sources are used, and give one example of an exercise. (411)

System	When in use	Examples of an exercise
ATP		
phosphocreatine		
anaerobic glycolysis		
aerobic glycolysis		
aerobic fat utilization		
aerobic protein utilization		

C. 1. "Anyone who exercises regularly, including the dieter, needs to consume a diet that includes moderate to high amounts of carbohydrates." Use Figure 11-6 to design a day's meal pattern that is high in carbohydrates. Then convert 55% of total kilocalories to grams of carbohydrates. If you are male, base 55% on a 3000 kcal diet; if you are female, use a 2500 kcal diet. Using Appendix A or the NutriTrac software, add up the number of grams as carbohydrates in each food choice. Does it exceed the number of grams you calculated as a goal in your diet? In addition, how does your diet compare to those shown in Table 11-4 (416)?

2. "Undertaking a carbohydrate-loading regimen is often advantageous to undertake to maximize muscle glycogen stores." Briefly describe carbohydrate loading: the process, what is the expected result, and a potential disadvantage. (418)

3. "A preevent meal should consist primarily of carbohydrate (about 70% of energy: 70 to 175 grams or more), have little dietary fiber, and include a moderate amount of fat and protein." Give an example of a preevent and postevent meal, including when the meal should be eaten. (422)

Preevent meal	Activity	Postevent meal
Time:	Time:	Time:

D. "Typical protein-intake recommendations for athletes range from 1.2 to 1.6 grams of protein per kilogram of body weight, considerably higher than the RDA of 0.8 grams per kilogram" (419). First calculate the number of grams of protein you would need (recall 2.2 pounds = 1 kilogram). Then indicate several protein-containing foods that would meet this requirement. (See Figure 7-8 or Appendix A in your textbook for excellent protein sources.)

E. "Athletes, especially female and adolescent athletes, should pay special attention to their iron intake." Review the advice provided for athletes for both iron and calcium intake in the textbook. Highlight some major points below. (420)

Iron:

Calcium:

F. "Athletes need this and generally even more water to maintain the body's ability to regulate its internal temperature and keep itself cool." Outline how sweating regulates body temperature and why fluid replacement is necessary. (423)

What is the general rule for timing and amount of fluid replacement during endurance athletic activities?

V. Applying nutrition to your life

"Moderate physical activity can improve your health and your chance of living longer. The best news is that you do not have to work out like a world-class athlete to reap most of the benefits. 'No pain-no gain' does not apply -- a moderate approach suffices" (402). A basic program should consist of a warm-up exercise, an exercise to increase muscular strength, endurance and flexibility, and finally a cool-down exercise. Design your own program for one week. Include warm-up (stretching), exercise activity and length, measurement of heart rate, and cool-down exercise. Then track your exercise and related fluid intake for the next week.

<u>Warm-up and cool-down</u>

Monday

Tuesday

Wednesday

Thursday

Friday

Saturday

Sunday

Activity	Typical heart rate	Time exercised	Fluid intake (cups)
Monday			
Tuesday			
Wednesday			
Thursday			
Friday			
Saturday			
Sunday			
	Average heart rate (total/7) _________	Average time (total/7) _________	Average cups (total/7) ______

How much total water or fluid did you generally drink before, after, and during exercise? Was this enough fluid to minimize fatigue and keep body weight approximately constant?

VI. Chapter 11 summary

Fill in the blanks using the words listed at the end of this summary.

Regular ______ activity is a vital part of a healthy lifestyle, constituting a total of at least ____ minutes per day of aerobic and resistance activities. People over _____ years should first discuss plans with a physician. Physically-active people show lower risks of premature heart disease, ______, and other common _____ diseases.

___________ is the major form of energy for cellular metabolism. All energy available to humans comes from ___________ energy. Plants capture solar energy using ___________. Human metabolic pathways are able to extract that energy from foodstuffs and ___________ it into ATP energy. _________ can also provide the energy needed to reform ATP.

In ___________, glucose is broken down into three-carbon compounds, yielding some ATP. The three-carbon compounds can then proceed to the ___________ pathway to form carbon dioxide and ___________ or an anaerobic pathway to form ___________ acid.

At low workloads, muscle cells mostly use ___________ for fuel. For intense exercise of short duration, muscles use the ___________ for energy. For more sustained high output activity, muscle glycogen breaks down and enters the glycolytic pathway, forming lactic acid. For endurance exercise, fat and carbohydrate are used as ___________; carbohydrate is used increasingly as activity intensifies. Little ___________ is used to fuel muscles.

Anyone who exercises needs to consume a diet that is moderate to high in ___________ and which follows the suggestions of the ___________. Vitamin and mineral supplements are indicated when ________ energy intakes make it difficult to meet ________ needs. Carbohydrate loading can ______________ the usual stores of muscle ___________. Participants in endurance events lasting more than ___________ hours benefit most from carbohydrate loading. This utilizes a diet containing ___________ amounts of carbohydrate for about 3 days before the event. Athletes should consume enough _________ to approximately maintain body weight during exercise. A ___________________ drink can be helpful for endurance athletes.

Use the following words to complete the summary:

aerobic	glycogen	photosynthesis
ATP	glycolysis	physical
carbohydrate	high	protein
chronic	increase	sports-type
convert	lactic	solar
diabetes	low	water
fat	nutrient	30
fluid	phosphocreatine (PCr)	35
Food Guide Pyramid	phosphocreatine system	2
fuel		

Check your answers using the summary for Chapter 11 in your textbook.

VII. Practice examination

Cover the answers on your initial attempt.

__B__ 1. The process in which plants use solar energy to produce carbohydrates is known as:

A. glycolysis.
B. photosynthesis.
C. citric acid cycle.
D. none of the above.

__D__ 2. The special form of energy used by cells is called:

A. ADP.
B. phosphocreatine.
C. glucose.
D. ATP.

__B__ 3. When glucose is broken down in a situation where oxygen supply is limited, a 3-carbon component known as ______________ accumulates in the muscle.

A. glycogen
B. lactic acid
C. phosphocreatine
D. nitrogen

__C__ 4. When there is plenty of oxygen available in the muscles, the condition is referred to as being:

A. anaerobic.
B. oxygenated.
C. aerobic.
D. ventilated.

__A__ 5. What is the major disadvantage of accumulating lactic acid in the muscles?

A. fatigue.
B. muscle damage.
C. nausea.
D. none -- it's an advantage.

__B__ 6. What is the preferable fuel for anaerobic glycolysis in an activity lasting less than two hours?

A. fatty acid
B. glycogen
C. blood glucose
D. amino acids

C 7. Athletes sometimes take carnitine pills in order to __________. However, this is of no value.

A. provide glycogen stones
B. build muscles
C. burn fat faster
D. increase foot speed

B 8. What source of energy is mainly used in light, aerobic activity?

A. carbohydrate
B. fat
C. protein
D. all of the above

D 9. Which of the foods below constitutes the best choice when one attempts carbohydrate loading before endurance events?

A. potato chips
B. french fries
C. all bran (high-fiber) cereal
D. rice

C 10. During muscle building regimens, athletes should consume how many grams of protein per kilogram of body weight?

A. 0.5 to 0.7 grams per kilograms.
B. 0.8 grams per kilograms.
C. 1 to 1.6 grams per kilograms.
D. 2 grams per kilograms.

B 11. During training the recommended dietary allowances for vitamins are greatly increased.

A. True
B. False

D 12. It is a good idea, especially for adult women athletes, to have blood hemoglobin regularly checked for deficiency of what mineral?

A. calcium
B. potassium
C. copper
D. iron

C 13. There is a correlation between low density of spinal bone in athletic women and:

A. type of exercise.
B. weight.
C. lack of menstruation.
D. iron deficiency.

C 14. A light meal is best eaten how many hours before a sporting event?

A. 4 to 6 hours
B. immediately before to give a boost of energy
C. 2 to 4 hours
D. You should not eat on the day of a sports event.

C 15. Caffeine, along with __________, has a dehydrating effect on the body, so fluids containing them should not be part of any hydration plan for exercise.

A. sugared soft drinks
B. dairy products
C. alcohol
D. carbohydrate solutions

D 16. Which of the following items is considered to be the best ergogenic aid to increase athletic performance?

A. bee pollen
B. salt tablets
C. coenzyme Q 10
D. none of the above

B 17. An ergogenic aid that is used in order to control lactic acid buildup in muscle is:

A. caffeine.
B. bicarbonate.
C. anabolic steroid.
D. growth hormone.

Chapter 12
Charting A Course for Change

I. Points to consider

Chapter 12 is designed to allow you to:

1. Outline the behavior change process.
2. Describe how to set goals and develop contracts to help meet these goals.
3. List how to modify habits and environments to encourage desired behavior changes.
4. State techniques to prevent behavior change relapse.
5. List some techniques for dining defensively.
6. Evaluate the pros and cons of "eating on the run."
7. Compare and contrast various traditional foods in several ethnic diets.

II. Word parts

Complete the following exercise using words in Chapter 12.

Word part	Meaning	Examples
arthr	joint	________________
psych	organ of thought and reason	________________
gno	to know	________________
lapse	to slip or fall back	________________

III. Flash cards

Cut out and review the flash cards for this chapter in Appendix A.

IV. Review and synthesis

A. "Behavior patterns that have evolved throughout a lifetime do not change or disappear overnight. Planned behavior changes occur gradually and with some effort." Briefly describe five steps in behavior change. (436)

a.

b.

c.

d.

e.

B. "Having decided to attempt a change, you begin a trial run." Outline the benefits and costs for changing one of your "problem" food behaviors. (438)

Benefits of changing the behavior.	Costs of changing the behavior.
Benefits of not changing the behavior.	Costs of not changing the behavior.

C. "The way to break the chain is to first identify the activities, pinpoint the weak links, break those links, and substitute other behaviors." Identify the links that make up one of your "problem" behaviors on the following diagram. Draw a line through the chain where it might be interrupted. Then add a link at that spot to fasten the beginning of a better outcome to the initial stimulus. Briefly describe the new desired outcome. (448)

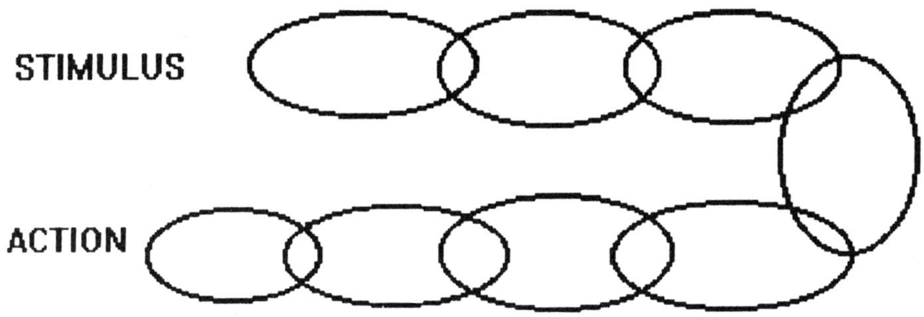

D. "Recruit support from others -- have some family members, roommates, or friends witness your contract; educate them about the program and your needs." Outline four tips that could help you prepare to change a problem food behavior. (449)

a.

b.

c.

d.

E. "Relapse often starts with a high-risk situation. Most people at first don't recognize the conditions that promote the relapse. One 'slip' sometimes snowballs into a series of lapses that lead to complete reversion into old behaviors." How do you think relapse into previous food habits is best minimized? Describe four methods. (450)

a.

b.

c.

d.

V. Applying nutrition to your life

"Once you establish goals and discover personal strengths and weaknesses in pursuing them, it's time to work out the details of the plan." List some tactics you could use for managing your "problem" food behaviors in the following situations. (442)

Buying and storing food

a.

b.

Cooking, preparing, and serving food

a.

b.

Eating food

a.

b.

Eating out in restaurants

a.

b.

Coping with emotions

a.

b.

VI. Chapter 12 summary

Fill in the blanks using the words listed at the end of this summary.

Behavior change occurs in a progression of steps. First, you become _______ of a problem. Then you openly receive new information about it, evolving a _______________ for learning. You undertake a _______ for the change, during which time positive reinforcement is critical. If an initial trial is successful, you may permanently ______ new behaviors. Before charting a behavior plan, it is important to identify your __________ regarding the behavior. A ______ could be kept at least for a week. This may show eating patterns and other behaviors that either contribute to or discourage new behaviors. This also helps reveal areas of the outside environment that need to be altered to reduce temptation.

When setting goals for a behavior plan, it is best to focus on _______ that lead to an intended result. Building ________ into the plan helps maintain momentum. After setting a plan of action, it is often helpful to develop a ________ that lists the actions intended to occur, the rewards to be received, and the ______ for the behavior change. The contract should at first reward positive ______ and later reward ultimate objectives. Before embarking on a behavior change program, the person should evaluate personal ______. A plan, no matter how skillfully developed, will not succeed unless a person has a strong desire to achieve the ________.

When implementing a plan, you need to monitor ________. Controlling your _________ can reduce temptations to deviate from the plan. Small _____ should be expected and not be seen as an excuse to abandon change. A __________ attitude can prevent collapse of the whole strategy. You need to plan for the possibility of _____. Most people revert to old behaviors during periods of stress or interpersonal conflict. Identify problem behavior chains and devise ways to substitute stronger for ______ links. Strategies to recover from relapse include identifying ________ situations in advance and mentally rehearsing a ________.

Choosing __________ foods is not so difficult in many of today's quick service restaurants. Some restaurants have evolved beyond hamburgers, French fries and milk shakes to include a variety of vegetables, ________, and ethnic foods. Still, ______ of the energy content in most quick service choices come from _________. Thus many of these meal selections are high calorie options when compared to the amount of other nutrients provided. A close look at fat intake and use of the _________ aids in making wise food choices.

Use the following words to complete the summary:

adopt	Food Guide Pyramid	rewards
aware	forgive-and forget	salad bars
behaviors	goals	small steps
commitment	healthy	strengths and weaknesses
contract	high-risk	time frame
environment	progress	trial period
failures	receptive framework	weaker
fat	relapse	40% to 50%
food diary	response	

Check your answers using the summary for Chapter 12 in your textbook; use page 146 of this Study Guide for the last five answers.

VII. Practice examination

Cover the answers on your initial attempt.

B 1. Behavior change:

A. is mostly a matter of willpower.
B. depends on a well-considered plan.
C. usually happens spontaneously.
D. requires the help of a professional.

D 2. Which of the following should be included in a food diary?

A. time of day
B. foods eaten and amount
C. mood
D. all of the above

A 3. The best way to make a behavior change is to:

A. attempt a series of small changes leading to the goal.
B. address the entire problem at once.
C. wait until your current behavior is dangerous.
D. set lofty goals.

D 4. The first step in the behavior change process is:

A. self-criticism.
B. adaptation.
C. trial change.
D. awareness.

C 5. Success at changing a behavior depends on:

A. the nature of the problem.
B. willpower.
C. commitment.
D. strategy.

B 6. Actual food choices are primarily determined by:

A. cost.
B. sensory appeal.
C. health value.
D. convenience.

D 7. A good plan for behavior change should:

A. focus on specific, measurable goals.
B. include appropriate rewards along the way.
C. allow for revision as needed.
D. all of the above.

C 8. Distorting information and denying facts to support wishful thinking is defined as:

A. behavior chains.
B. contingency management.
C. rationalization.
D. positive reinforcement.

D 9. If a lapse occurs:

A. realize that you are only human and plan to prevent other lapses.
B. it is an indication that your plan is unsuccessful.
C. it may be an indication of stress or internal conflict.
D. A and C

D 10. Eating patterns are difficult to change because:

A. eating is closely tied to social occasions.
B. people eat not only for hunger but for pleasure.
C. people may use food to fight boredom, stress, or loneliness.
D. all of the above.

D 11. Which one of the following cooking techniques does not promote less fat?

A. broiling.
B. stir-frying.
C. roasting.
D. breading.

B 12. Quick service foods are often high in ________, and so choices should be made carefully.

A. carbohydrate
B. fat
C. protein
D. dietary fiber

D 13. Behavior modification is defined as:

A. recognizing which foods are high in calories.
B. accepting the fact that people are fat because of a genetic predisposition.
C. accepting psychological counseling for eating problems.
D. finding ways to modify behaviors that contribute to health problems.

A 14. Forming a plan of action to respond to environmental conditions when overeating is likely is designated by weight-loss professionals as:

A. contingency management.
B. self-monitoring.
C. stimulus control.
D. restraint.

Answers to selected questions

VI. healthy; salad bars; 40% to 50%; fat; Food Guide Pyramid

Chapter 13
Anorexia Nervosa and Bulimia Nervosa

I. Points to consider

Chapter 13 is designed to allow you to:

1. Contrast healthy attitudes toward uses of food with behavior patterns that could lead to unhealthy uses of food.
2. Outline the causes of, effects of, typical persons affected by, and treatment for anorexia nervosa.
3. Outline the causes of, effects of, typical persons affected by, and treatment for bulimia nervosa.
4. Outline the causes of, effects of, typical persons affected by, and treatment for binge eating disorder.
5. Relate the existence of eating disorders to current social trends.
6. Describe methods to reduce the development of eating disorders, including the use of early warning signs to identify early cases.

II. Word parts

Complete the following exercise using words in Chapter 13.

Word part	Meaning	Examples
or	mouth	____________
lim	hunger	____________
kal	potassium	____________
bar	weight	____________
lan	wool	____________
syn	with, together	____________
bary	heavy	____________

III. Flash cards

Cut out and review the flash cards for this chapter in Appendix A.

IV. Review and synthesis

A. "In our society, we are bombarded daily with images of the 'ideal' body. Television programs, billboard advertisements, magazine pictures, movies and newspapers tell us that an ultra-slim body will bring happiness, love, and even success." (461)

1. Name two media examples that influenced you to think or act in a different way, and how, if taken to the extreme, these influences could be destructive.

    a.

    b.

2. Name three constructive and healthy ways (related to food) that you personally can work toward a happy, successful life.

    a.

    b.

    c.

B. "Anorexia nervosa may begin as a simple attempt to lose weight. A comment from a well-meaning friend, relative, or coach suggesting that the person seems to be gaining weight or is too fat may be all that is needed." Complete the following table. Keep in mind these eating disorders often overlap, but ignore that for now. (465)

	Societal pressures that may trigger disease	Physical symptoms	Psychological traits
Anorexia nervosa			
Bulimia nervosa			

C. "A person with anorexia nervosa refuses to eat enough. This refusal is the hallmark of the disease, whether or not other practices such as binge-purge cycles appear." Sally is a 19-year old college sophomore with a 7-year history of anorexia nervosa. She is 5 feet, 7 inches tall and weighs 90 pounds. List six of the possible physical effects of anorexia nervosa on her. (466)

a.

b.

c.

d.

e.

f.

D. 1. "Susceptible people may have both biological factors and lifestyle patterns that predispose them to becoming overweight." From what you know about the physiology and characteristics of obesity, describe three possible predisposing factors for bulimia nervosa. (471)

a.

b.

c.

2. Add to this list three societal factors that can increase the risk for development of bulimia nervosa. (390)

a.

b.

c.

E. "The person with bulimia nervosa may think of food constantly. In contrast to the anorexic person who turns away from food when faced with problems, the bulimic person turns toward food in critical situations." Do your life situations affect your response to food, causing you to eat either more or less than usual? Name three alternative coping mechanisms you could use at these times (consult Chapter 10 if needed). (471)

a.

b.

c.

F. "Among sufferers of bulimia nervosa, bingeing often alternates with attempts to rigidly restrict food intake." Explain the process (or cycle) of bingeing and purging. (471)

G. "Binge-eating disorder is most likely to develop in people who never learned to appropriately express and deal with their feelings. Rather than face their problems, they turn to food instead." Although it is also classified as an eating disorder, how does binge-eating disorder in general differ from bulimia nervosa and anorexia nervosa? (477)

What are two ways people with binge eating disorder can help overcome their disorder?

a.

b.

V. Applying nutrition to your life

"The American College of Sports Medicine (ACSM) has named the syndrome consisting of disordered eating, lack of menstrual periods, and compromised bone density the female athlete triad." You suspect that your close friend has an eating disorder. (476)

1. How might you approach that person with your concerns?

2. What steps could you take to aid that person in getting professional help and during treatment?

3. Who else can help you with this situation? Why?

4. Is there any place on your campus or in the surrounding community where a person can receive help with such an eating disorder? If yes, where is it located? If no, investigate further, since most communities have these resources.

VI. Chapter 13 summary

Fill in the blanks using the words listed at the end of this summary.

The person with anorexia nervosa is usually a girl around the age of ________ who begins to diet but then finds it difficult to stop. The person is generally a _________ and high achiever. Early warning signs for anorexia nervosa include abnormal food habits, such as cooking a meal but refusing to eat it or classifying foods as _______ and unsafe. Later, the person often ______ from family and friends and develops a very _______ and joyless nature.

Physical effects of anorexia nervosa include a decrease in body temperature and ______, iron deficiency ______, a low white blood cell count, hair loss, constipation, low blood ________, and the cessation of ___________. Treatment of anorexia nervosa includes increasing food intake to at least an amount sufficient to support _________ weight gain. Psychological counseling attempts to help patients establish ______ food habits and find means of coping with the _________ that led to the disorder. _________ may be necessary.

Bulimia nervosa is characterized by _________ on large amounts of food at one sitting and then _________ by _________, _________ use, exercise, or other means. Both men and women are at risk. Vomiting as a means of purging is especially destructive to the body: it can cause severe _________, stomach ulcers, irritation of the esophagus, low blood potassium, and other problems. Bulimia nervosa poses a serious health problem and is associated with significant risk of _______.

Treatment of bulimia nervosa includes ___________ as well as nutritional counseling. During treatment, the person learns to ___________ himself or herself and cope with problems in ways which do not involve ___________. Regular ___________ patterns are developed as the bulimic person begins to plan meals in an informed, ___________ manner.

The female athlete triad, consisting of disordered ______, lack of menstrual periods, and abnormally low _______, is particularly seen in appearance-related and endurance sports. If not corrected, this disorder will eventually lead to decreased athletic performance and general health problems.

_________, which is more widespread than either anorexia nervosa or bulimia nervosa, is most common among people with a history of frequent, unsuccessful ______. Binge eaters typically either practice _________ (i.e., eating continually over extended periods) or bingeing without purging. ________ disturbances are often at the root of this disordered form of eating. Treatment addresses deeper emotional issues, discourages food _________ and restrictive diets, and helps to restore normal _________.

___________ is a condition where children are ___________ by parents in an attempt to limit risk of future disease, such as ______________ or heart disease. Growth failure -- reduced weight and height gains -- can result if ___________ intake is not increased to appropriate amounts.

___________ has been ranked as the most dreaded deviation from our cultural ideals of body image. Over the course of this century, a woman's "ideal" body form has become ___________. Researchers have linked this preference for a ___________ body type to the recent surge in __________________.

Use the following words to complete the summary:

accept	eating (2x)	laxative	purging
anemia	eating behaviors	lean	regular
baryophobia	eating disorders	life stresses	safe
binge-eating disorder	emotional	menstrual periods	slow
bingeing	fatness	nutrient	suicide
bone density	food	obesity	thinner
critical	grazing	perfectionist	tooth decay
deprivation	healthful	potassium	underfed
dieting	heart rate	psychological	vomiting
	hospitalization	puberty	withdraws

Check your answers using the summary for Chapter 13 in your textbook; use page 154 of this Study Guide for the last four answers.

VII. Practice examination

Cover the answers on your initial attempt.

__A__ 1. A long-term health consequence of anorexia nervosa could be:

A. fractures resulting from bone loss.
B. atherosclerotic heart disease.
C. infertility.
D. cancer.

__B__ 2. An early warning sign of anorexia nervosa is:

A. hoarding food.
B. withdrawal from family.
C. secret bingeing.
D. use of ipecac syrup.

__A__ 3. The major health risk from frequent vomiting from bulimia nervosa is:

A. a potassium imbalance.
B. constipation.
C. lanugo.
D. swollen glands.

For questions 4 to 13 indicate which of the following characteristics are mainly associated with anorexia nervosa (A), and which are mainly associated with bulimia nervosa (B). Ignore that some characteristics may be associated with both eating disorders.

__A__ 4. Intense fear of becoming obese.

__B__ 5. Awareness of abnormal eating pattern.

__A__ 6. Distorted image of body size.

__B__ 7. Depressed mood following binges.

__B__ 8. May be above healthy weight for height.

A 9. Fear of not being able to stop eating.

A 10. Loss of menses.

A 11. Refusal to maintain body weight within normal limits.

B 12. Secretive eating.

A 13. Compulsive physical activity.

C 14. Which of the following does not describe people suffering from starvation?

A. state of extreme weakness and collapse
B. mental disorientation
C. hyperactive, hungry, and actively clamoring for food
D. extreme apathy and indifference

D 15. Anorexia nervosa is a disease primarily affecting:

A. children.
B. elderly women.
C. young boys.
D. teenage women.

C 16. The most successful treatment for anorexia nervosa involves:

A. isolation from the family and forced tube feeding.
B. dietary counseling on an outpatient basis by a registered dietitian.
C. inpatient psychological, nutritional, and medical therapy, often involving the whole family.
D. use of diuretics.

C 17. A critical goal in the early stages of the treatment of a person with anorexia nervosa is to:

A. increase the patient's weight to her goal body weight within the first month.
B. establish regular meal patterns.
C. allow the person a feeling of control over her life.
D. get the patient to realize how unbecoming her body has become.

D 18. Bulimic patients often have a problem with:

A. recognizing nutritious food choices.
B. eating enough food to maintain a healthy body weight.
C. obesity.
D. an inability to control responses to impulse and desire.

B 19. Characteristics of a person exhibiting binge-eating disorder often include:

A. a persistent concern with body shape, weight, and thinness.
B. regularly eating to avoid feeling and dealing with emotional pain.
C. family history with a constrictive internal structure.
D. adoption of rigid "food rules".

D 20. For a person with binge-eating disorder, food is used to:

A. reduce stress and avoid life problems.
B. produce feelings of power and well-being.
C. avoid feelings of intimacy with others.
D. all of the above.

Answers to selected questions

VI. fatness; thinner; lean; eating disorders

Chapter 14
Pregnancy and Breastfeeding

I. Points to consider

Chapter 14 is designed to allow you to:

1. List major changes occurring in the body during pregnancy and the altered nutrient needs associated with each change.
2. List factors that may interfere with a successful pregnancy outcome.
3. Specify the optimal weight gain during pregnancy for the normal adult woman.
4. Plan an adequate, balanced diet for the pregnant woman and the breastfeeding woman using the Food Guide Pyramid as a basis.
5. Identify the nutrients that may need to be supplemented during pregnancy and explain the reason for each.
6. Explain how typical discomforts of pregnancy may be minimized by diet changes.
7. Describe the physiology of breastfeeding and give some advantages of breastfeeding for the mother and infant.

II. Word parts

Complete the following exercise using words in Chapter 14.

Word part	Meaning	Examples
nat	to be born	______________
gest	to bear	______________
fet	offspring	______________
pica	magpie	______________
tri	three	______________
syn	together, with	______________

III. Flash cards

Cut out and review the flash cards for this chapter in Appendix A.

IV. Review and synthesis

A. "Although some aspects of fetal and newborn health are beyond our control, a woman's conscious decisions about social, health, and nutritional factors affect her infant's health and future." List three problems that may contribute to a higher risk during pregnancy. Briefly outline the mechanism for each. (492)

a.

b.

c.

B. "The RDA for protein increases by 10 to 15 grams daily, depending on age." The fetus needs nutrients for energy and the growth and development of tissues and organs. List two key nutrients associated with each of the following. Then list a good food source for each. (500)

Increased Need	Key Nutrient	Food Source
a. Protein synthesis	________	________
	________	________
b. Bone growth	________	________
	________	________
c. Energy metabolism	________	________
	________	________
d. Collagen formation	________	________
	________	________
e. Blood formation	________	________
	________	________

Check your answers using page 166 of this Study Guide.

C. "Researchers in Great Britain took this one step further. They showed that height and social class were better predictors than dietary intake during pregnancy." What are two possible consequences if a woman enters pregnancy in poor nutritional status? Postulate a reason for each. (505)

a.

b.

D. "Nutrient needs for a breastfeeding mother change slightly, if at all, from those of the pregnant woman." (517) Compare the RDA for the following nutrients for a pregnant woman with those for a lactating woman. (Use the inside cover of your textbook.)

NUTRIENT	A. Pregnant woman	B. Lactating woman	Difference (A - B)	Food choice to meet need	Amount of the nutrient present
Protein					
Vitamin A					
Vitamin D					
Thiamin					
Riboflavin					
Niacin					
Vitamin C					
Calcium					
Zinc					

Use Appendix A in your textbook to check whether the nutrient content of the potential food choices supply the increased needs you listed. See if just one or two food choices will suffice to meet all extra nutrient needs.

E. "One approach to a diet that supports a successful pregnancy is based on the Food Guide Pyramid." Outline the diet plan for pregnant women proposed in your textbook. Indicate approximate serving sizes. (502)

Food group	Number of servings	Specific food choices
Milk, yogurt, and cheese		
Meat, poultry, fish, dry beans, eggs, and nuts		
Vegetables		
Fruits		
Breads, cereals, rice, and pasta		

F. "She cannot afford a cheeseburger for herself and another for the fetus." In what way must a pregnant woman eat for two? Why? (497)

G. "The National Academy of Sciences supports the use of iron supplements but no other vitamin or mineral supplements during a routine pregnancy."

1. What three nutrients may be the focus of supplementation in the diet during pregnancy? Why? (502)

 a.

 b.

 c.

2. A total vegetarian (vegan) especially needs to carefully plan a diet for pregnancy. List four nutrient needs the pregnant vegan should pay special attention to based on the chapter discussion and what you recall from the Nutrition Issue in Chapter 7. Indicate a vegan food source for each.

   a.

   b.

   c.

   d.

See page 166 for possible answers.

H. "Although a mother's digestive and metabolic systems work very efficiently, some discomfort accompanies the changes her body undergoes to accommodate the fetus." List four common complaints of pregnancy that may be related to diet. Briefly indicate how to try to solve each problem. (509)

   a.

   b.

   c.

   d.

I. 1. "Human milk is tailored to meet infant nutrient needs for the first 4 to 6 months of life. The possible exceptions are fluoride, iron, and vitamin D." Compare and contrast use of human milk and commercial infant formulas. (518)

Factors	Human milk	Commercial formula
Prevention of infections		
Risk of contamination		
Risk of allergies		
Convenience		

2. "Although formula feeding can satisfy the infant, breastfeeding offers many physiological advantages." Breastfeeding benefits both the mother and infant. What are three potential benefits not listed in Part 1 for either the mother or the infant? (518)

a.

b.

c.

V. Applying nutrition to your life

A. "Breastfeeding reduces the general risk of infections to the infant." If you were asked to conduct a class for pregnant women on the benefits of breastfeeding, what 4 main points would you highlight during this session? (518)

a.

b.

c.

d.

B. How would you answer the following questions?

a. How can I continue to breastfeed when I am at work?

b. Is it OK to have a glass of wine at dinner while I'm breastfeeding?

c. How old should my baby be when I begin to wean him or her from the breast?

d. Is it OK to diet while I'm breastfeeding?

e. How do I know if my infant is getting enough milk?

VI. Chapter 14 summary

Fill in the blanks using the words listed at the end of this summary.

Adequate nutrition is vital during pregnancy to ensure the well-being of both the infant and the mother. Problems caused by poor nutrition and some medications can cause _________, especially in the first trimester. Growth retardation and altered development are possible if insults occur later in pregnancy. Infants born ________ (before 37 weeks of gestation) or with low ________ (less than 5.5 pounds, or 2500 grams) usually have more medical problems at birth than do normal infants.

Daily energy needs increase by an average of ______ kcal during the last two trimesters of pregnancy. Weight gain should occur slowly, reaching a total of ______ pounds in a woman at healthy body weight. Protein, vitamin, and mineral requirements increase with pregnancy. Extra servings from the _________ and the meat, poultry, fish, dry beans, eggs, and nuts group of the __________________ are recommended. _______ and folate in particular may need to be supplemented in the diet. ______ pregnancy requires very careful prenatal and nutritional care. Complications occur more often in these pregnancies because of the very high _______ demands and often poor social and economic support.

Pregnancy-induced hypertension, ______, constipation, nausea and vomiting, edema, and ______ are all possible complications of pregnancy. Nutrition therapy can often help minimize these problems.

Almost all women have the ability to nurse their infants. The nutrient composition of human milk is very different from unaltered ________________. The first fluid, called __________, is very rich in _________. Advantages of breastfeeding over formula-feeding for the infant include fewer intestinal, respiratory, and ear ________, as well as fewer infant ______ and intolerances. An infant can be adequately nourished with formula if the mother chooses not to breastfeed.

Breastfeeding is not desirable if the mother has certain diseases or must take _______ that is potentially harmful to the infant.

_________ is one potential energy source that should be avoided during pregnancy. _______ are commonly seen in infants exposed to high amounts _________. More subtle defects in development are suspected at lower intakes.

Use the following words to complete the summary:

alcohol	Food Guide Pyramid	milk, yogurt, and cheese group
allergies	heartburn	psychological
anemia	immune factors	preterm
birth defects (2x)	infections	teenage
birth weight	in utero	25 to 35
colostrum	iron	300
cow's milk	medication	

Check your answers using the summary for Chapter 14 in your textbook; use page 166 of this Study Guide for the last three answers.

VII. Practice examination

Cover the answers on your initial attempt.

__D__ 1. Which of the following mothers probably faces the highest pregnancy risk?

A. white, mature, lower socioeconomic family
B. adolescent, nonwhite, upper middle-class family
C. white, mature, middle-class family
D. adolescent, nonwhite, lower socioeconomic family

__B__ 2. The pregnant woman needs to increase her energy intake by about ______ per day during the last two trimesters of pregnancy.

A. 100 kcal
B. 300 kcal
C. 500 kcal
D. 800 kcal

__C__ 3. The breastfeeding woman with normal fat stores from pregnancy needs to increase her energy intake by about ______ per day.

A. 100 kcal
B. 300 kcal
C. 500 kcal
D. 800 kcal

__D__ 4. Which of the following is not an attribute of human milk?

A. lactose content
B. presence of a bifidus factor
C. antibody content
D. high mineral content

__D__ 5. The hormone responsible for the let-down reflex in breastfeeding is:

A. thyroid-stimulating hormone.
B. prolactin.
C. insulin.
D. oxytocin.

__C__ 6. Which of the following is not a component of weight gain in pregnancy?

A. breast tissue
B. amniotic fluid
C. thigh muscles
D. blood volume

__D__ 7. An energy source to avoid in pregnancy is:

A. fat.
B. protein.
C. carbohydrate.
D. alcohol.

__B__ 8. Weight gain in pregnancy should usually be at least about:

A. 15 to 20 pounds. B. 25 to 35 pounds. C. 30 to 40 pounds. D. 35 to 45 pounds.

__B__ 9. A major advantage of breastfeeding for the infant is:

A. the E. coli factor.
B. passive immunity.
C. the high casein content.
D. low lactose content.

__B__ 10. Colostrum:

A. can be synthesized by the newborn infant but not by a fetus.
B. is a source of antibodies and secreted from the breast for the first few days after birth.
C. contains mainly fat.
D. is a hormone involved in stimulating lactation.

B 11. It is often recommended that breastfed infants be supplemented with which of the following nutrients?

A. iron and vitamin B-6
B. vitamin D and iron
C. calcium and iron
D. vitamin C and vitamin D

C 12. The fetus receives nourishment primarily through:

A. antibodies.
B. meconium.
C. the placenta.
D. amniotic fluid.

B 13. During pregnancy the woman who is a vegan may not obtain adequate amounts of which of the following nutrients?

A. niacin, vitamin D, magnesium, and iodide
B. calcium, iron, zinc, and vitamin B-12
C. thiamin, niacin, riboflavin, and folate
D. vitamin C, vitamin B-6, phosphorus, and sodium

D 14. An attribute of human milk that keeps the infant from supporting the growth of some harmful intestinal bacteria is:

A. lactase.
B. albumin.
C. let-down reflex.
D. bifidus factor.

A 15. In general, nutritional deficits in the breastfeeding mother:

A. reduce the quantity of her milk.
B. reduce all nutrients equally.
C. stop lactation entirely.
D. reduce the quality of her milk.

C 16. The let-down reflex:

A. causes depression in a new mother after the birth.
B. moves the hindmilk toward the nipple after the infant has drawn the foremilk.
C. forces milk to the nipple area of the breast.
D. makes a newborn turn toward whichever cheek is touched and search for the nipple.

C 17. An increased requirement for ________ during pregnancy is related to their roles in the synthesis of red blood cells.

A. vitamin E and vitamin C
B. iron and vitamin K
C. folate and vitamin B-12
D. protein and calcium

A 18. The "physiological anemia of pregnancy" is a result of a(n):

A. increase in the mother's blood volume.
B. decrease in the mother's iron absorption.
C. decrease in the mother's water consumption.
D. decrease in the mother's red blood cell production.

D 19. A maternal practice that can be harmful to the fetus is:

A. a low-carbohydrate diet.
B. fasting.
C. smoking.
D. all of the above.

D 20. To produce a healthy infant, the mother should ideally have an adequate diet:

A. during the 9 months she carries the infant.
B. during the last trimester when the baby is growing so rapidly.
C. during the second and third trimesters of pregnancy.
D. beginning months before conception occurs and continuing through the period of lactation.

D 21. Select the following factor that is least likely to pose a risk to maternal and fetal health during pregnancy and childbirth.

A. underweight mother
B. maternal age 15 years or under
C. many closely spaced pregnancies
D. maternal age of 30 to 35 years

B 22. To avoid constipation, the pregnant woman should increase her intake of:

A. milk and dairy products.
B. whole-grain bread and fruits.
C. sugars and starches.
D. lean meat, poultry, and fish.

C 23. The practice of eating dirt, clay, or laundry starch during pregnancy is called:

A. meconium.
B. cretinism.
C. pica.
D. pregnancy-induced hypertension.

D 24. Advantages and benefits of breastfeeding to the mother include all but which of the following?

A. greater convenience
B. a more rapid loss of the fat tissue that may have accumulated in her body during pregnancy
C. fosters close contact between mother and infant
D. less nutritional demands on the mother

B 25. Infants born after normal gestation length but weighing less than 5½ pounds are labeled:

A. low birth weight.
B. small for gestational age.
C. premature.
D. normal, the smaller the better.

Answers to selected questions

IV. B.
a. vitamin B-6 and amino acids -- chicken meets both needs
b. calcium and vitamin D -- fortified milk meets both needs
c. thiamin and riboflavin -- enriched breads meets both needs
d. vitamin C -- oranges; amino acids -- chicken
e. iron -- beef; folate -- spinach
f. potassium and vitamin A -- apricots meet both needs

G.2. calcium, vitamin D, iron, zinc. See Chapters 8 and 9 if you need to identify good food sources.

VI. alcohol; birth defects; in utero

Chapter 15
Nutrition From Infancy Through Adolescence

I. Points to consider

Chapter 15 is designed to allow you to:

1. Describe how nutrition affects infant growth and physiological development.
2. Outline the diet guidelines to meet the basic nutritional needs for normal growth and development for the infant and discuss some do's and don'ts associated with infant feeding.
3. List several challenges parents must face in dealing with childhood eating habits.
4. List the nutrients often found to be lacking in the diet of infants, toddlers, preschoolers, and teenagers and make recommendations to remedy the problems.
5. Distinguish between food allergies and intolerances and make recommendations for treating both.

II. Word parts

Complete the following exercise using words in Chapter 15.

Word part	Meaning	Examples
pharmac	related to a medicine or drug	____________
plas	to form	____________
troph	nutrition	____________
arche	beginning	____________
andr	male	____________
gen	produce	____________
cyto	cell	____________

III. Flash cards

Cut out and review the flash cards for this chapter in Appendix A.

IV. Review and synthesis

A. "From observations of Egyptian mummies, we see that infants were about the same size in 300 BC as they are today. However, adult mummies are much smaller than adults today." (530)

1. Nutrient needs increase during the first year of life. For the following nutrients, describe one function in relation to growth and development.

	Nutrients	Function
a.	protein	____________________
b.	vitamin A	____________________
c.	vitamin C	____________________
d.	vitamin D	____________________
e.	iron	____________________
f.	calcium	____________________
g.	zinc	____________________

See Chapters 7, 8, and 9 in your textbook if you need to refresh your memory.

2. What two general criteria would you use for selecting an infant formula for <u>your</u> healthy infant? (538)

   a.

   b.

B. "A common reason offered for introducing solid foods early--before 4 to 6 months of age -- is the belief that it helps the infant sleep through the night. However, many studies have shown that sleeping through the night is a developmental milestone for the infant." (543)

1. Discuss three reasons why solid foods are not recommended for an infant during the first few months of life.

   a.

   b.

   c.

2. Describe one approach for the introduction of semisolid foods and table foods in infancy.

	Age (months)		
	4 to 6	6 to 8	9 to 12

In the boxes, put foods to start at the ages indicated.

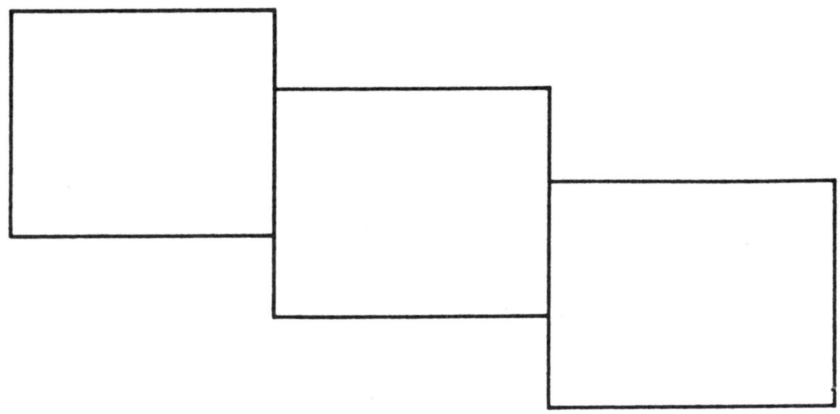

C. "In response to various controversies surrounding infant feeding, the American Academy of Pediatrics has issued a number of statements concerning infant diets." What current recommendations would you give parents concerning the use of fat, cholesterol, salt, and sugar in the diet of an infant? (539)

a. Fat

b. Cholesterol

c. Salt

d. Sugar

D. "The rapid growth rate that characterizes infancy tapers off quickly during the subsequent few years. The average annual weight gain is only 4.5 to 6.6 pounds between the ages of 2 and 5 years." A 2-year-old's mother is discussing the child's nutritional needs with you. The mother is concerned because the child is eating less than what her mother thinks the 2-year-old should be eating. She is gaining weight and growing normally, but the mother states that the child had a better appetite a year ago. Should this mother be concerned? Why or why not? (549)

E. "Surprisingly, children generally eat what they are offered. If given whole-grain breakfast cereals, whole-wheat bread, vegetables, salad, and fresh fruits regularly, young children accept most of these foods and eat them."

1. List four general guidelines to follow when planning diets for preschoolers. (550)

a.

b.

c.

d.

2. Outline a food plan for a 5-year-old girl, and then in the right-hand column develop a 1-day diet. (552)

Food group	Number of servings	Actual foods to help meet recommendation
Milk, yogurt, and cheese		
Meat, poultry, fish, dry beans, eggs, and nuts		
Vegetables		
Fruits		
Breads, cereals, rice, and pasta		

F. "For teenagers, it's more effective to focus on the benefits of healthful foods and regular physical activity they can reap right now than to talk about health hazards that may or may not happen at some later time."

1. Adolescents pose nutritional concerns as a result of their lifestyles. List three lifestyle characteristics that may jeopardize their nutritional status. (560)

a.

b.

c.

2. List the two potential advantages and disadvantages of snacking during the teen years. (562)

<u>Advantages</u>	<u>Disadvantages</u>
a.	a.
b.	b.

V. Applying nutrition to your life

"Major scientific groups, such as the American Dietetic Association and the American Society for Clinical Nutrition, believe that vitamin and mineral supplements are unnecessary for healthy children; it's better to emphasize good foods." (554) Find the listing of a school lunch menu in your local newspaper, or use the following one. Using your NutriTrac software or Appendix A in your textbook, do a nutritional analysis for the following nutrients for a 9-year-old boy you are baby-sitting for a week while his parents are in Europe.

Your menu	Sample lunch menu	Approximate serving size
	pepperoni pizza	4½ ounces (135 grams)
	chocolate chip cookie	3/4 ounce (21 grams)
	banana	1/2 of large size
	2% low-fat milk	1 cup

	Nutrient intake from meal	One third of RDA for 9-year-old boy
Energy (kcal)	______________	______________
Protein (g)	______________	______________
Vitamin A (RE)	______________	______________
Thiamin (mg)	______________	______________
Riboflavin (mg)	______________	______________
Vitamin C (mg)	______________	______________
Calcium (mg)	______________	______________
Iron (mg)	______________	______________

VI. Chapter 15 summary

Fill in the blanks using the words listed at the end of this summary.

Growth is very rapid during infancy; birth weight doubles in _________ months and length increases by ____________ in the first year. An adequate diet is very important to support normal growth. Undernutrition can cause irreversible changes in growth and development. Growth in infants and children can be assessed by measuring body weight, ________________ (or length), and head circumference over time. Nutrient needs in the first 6 months can be met by __________ or formula. Supplementary ___________ and iron may be needed in the first 6 months for breastfed infants, and supplemental ___________ may be needed by both breastfed and formula-fed infants.

Infant formulas generally contain lactose or sucrose, heat-treated proteins from cow's milk, and vegetable oil. These formulas may or may not be fortified with ______. Sanitation is very important in preparing and storing formula. For most infants this readiness for solid food occurs between 4 to 6 ______ of age. Solid food should not be added to an infant's diet until there is a __________, the gastrointestinal tract is able to digest these complex foods, the infant has the __________ to control tongue thrusting, and the risk of developing ______ has decreased. The first solid food given should be iron-fortified _________, with very gradual addition of other foods, one at a time per __________. Some foods to avoid giving infants in the first year include cow's milk (especially ________ varieties), very salty or sweet foods, or foods that may cause choking. Introduction of iron-containing solid food at the appropriate time and not offering ________ until 1 year of age can generally prevent _______ anemia in later infancy.

Obese children and adolescents are more likely to become obese ___________ and so incur greater health risks. Parents can provide healthful food choices, while ___________ should control portion sizes. When controlled early, a problem of obesity may ___________ as the child continues to grow in height. Obese _________, on the other hand, do not necessarily go on to become obese children.

A slower rate of growth in the preschool years makes the choice of _________ foods and a reduction in serving size important. Iron-rich foods, such as _________, are an important part of the Food Guide Pyramid at this age. Teens should focus on adequate iron and ___________ in the diet, and strive to moderate high _________ food choices.

___________ does not appear to be related to eating chocolate or any other specific foods. It is caused by overactive ___________ (sebaceous) glands that respond, in part, to high amounts of ___________ in the blood. Treatment options now include acutane, a ___________ derivative.

Food allergies may be caused by _________ responses to food. Elimination or a reduction in the use of allergy-causing foods can bring relief. ___________ an infant is a wise preventative step for future generations. Food _______ are not caused by allergic responses but rather by offending substances in foods, such as lactose in the presence of low intestinal lactase activity, or Salmonella bacteria toxins.

Use the following words to complete the summary:

acne	fat-secreting	infant cereals	physical ability
adults	fluoride	intolerances	self-correct
breastfeeding	food allergies	iron	testosterone
calcium	height	iron-deficiency	vitamin A
children	honey	lean red meats	vitamin D
cow's milk	human milk	months	week
fat	immune	nutrient-dense	4 to 6
fat-reduced	infants	nutritional need	50%

Check your answers using the summary for Chapter 15 in the textbook; use the next page of this Study Guide for the last seven answers.

Answers to selected questions

VI. acne; fat-secreting; testosterone; vitamin A; immune; breastfeeding; intolerances

VII. Practice examination

Cover the answers on your initial attempt.

__B__ 1. The first solid food(s) usually first added to the infant's diet is (are):

A. milk.
B. iron-fortified cereals.
C. fruits.
D. vegetables.

__C__ 2. Which of the following nutrients are needed for the synthesis of protein tissue in both the fetus and the newborn?

A. vitamin C, vitamin D, and niacin
B. vitamin A, copper, and calcium
C. vitamin B-6, vitamin B-12, and zinc
D. thiamin, niacin, and riboflavin

__C__ 3. During the late childhood and adolescent periods, the RDA are greatly increased for:

A. vitamin A, vitamin D, and calcium.
B. vitamin C, folate, and zinc.
C. calcium, phosphorus, and iron.
D. vitamin B-6, vitamin B-12, and folate.

__A__ 4. The nutrients most often deficient in the diets of American adolescents are:

A. calcium and iron.
B. protein and vitamin C.
C. thiamin and iron.
D. calcium and vitamin D.

__B__ 5. Obese children should strive to:

A. ignore their problem.
B. maintain their weight and "grow into it".
C. avoid salt.
D. first lose weight until it is more desirable for height.

__D__ 6. A newborn baby should triple his or her birth weight by about ______ of age?

A. 10 months
B. 6 months
C. 8 months
D. 12 months

__B__ 7. The cutoff for low-birth-weight babies is _____ kilograms.

A. 2.1
B. 2.5
C. 2.7
D. 2.3

__D__ 8. Most health authorities recommend that solid food should be given to the infant at what age?

A. 3 to 4 months
B. 1 month
C. 2 months
D. 4 to 6 months

C 9. When children are about 1 year of age, their appetite decreases. This is caused by:

A. dislike of foods served.
B. more interest in the environment.
C. decrease in growth rate.
D. loss of interest in food.

A 10. A good rule of thumb for feeding preschool children is _____ of each food served for each year of age.

A. 1 tablespoon
B. 2 tablespoons
C. 3 tablespoons
D. 4 tablespoons

B 11. Protein allowances for infants are about _____ per kilogram of body weight per day.

A. 1 gram
B. 2 grams
C. 4 grams
D. 8 grams

D 12. A food allergen can be identified by:

A. the child's likes and dislikes for foods.
B. noting the symptoms; milk causes a skin rash whereas chocolate causes diarrhea.
C. noting what was eaten at the last meal.
D. a trial of food elimination and a later challenge feeding of the suspected food.

C 13. Nutrients that may be low in infant vegetarian diets are:

A. folate and vitamin C.
B. vitamin A and vitamin C.
C. vitamin B-12 and zinc.
D. protein and thiamin.

C 14. Which of the following factors is NOT a predictor of child and adolescent obesity?

A. time spent watching television
B. family history of obesity
C. number of siblings
D. weight at 6 to 8 years of age

A 15. It is recommended that honey not be part of an infant's diet because it:

A. is linked to infant botulism.
B. is too high in energy content.
C. causes constipation.
D. has low bioavailability for glucose.

C 16. It is unwise to leave a bottle in the infant's mouth after he or she falls asleep because:

A. the infant will ingest too much sodium.
B. this practice may lead to obesity.
C. this practice may cause tooth decay.
D. this practice may cause tooth distortion.

D 17. The WIC program is primarily for:

A. pregnant women until delivery only.
B. school age children until age 7 years.
C. school age children until age 10 years.
D. pregnant women and children up to 5 years of age.

C 18. Fat-reduced milk is not recommended for children under _____ of age.

A. 6 months
B. 1 year
C. 2 years
D. 5 years

A 19. The major problem with fast foods for adolescents is that these are:

A. often high in fat and energy content and often low in calcium and fiber.
B. too expensive for the amount of nutritive value they contribute.
C. low in iron, thiamin, riboflavin, and niacin.
D. too high in sugar.

A 20. If a 1-year-old child wants to spoon-feed himself clumsily, the parent should:

A. let the child try so he or she will learn.
B. gently take the spoon away and feed him or her.
C. use behavior modification techniques.
D. let the child eat with his or her fingers instead.

D 21. The food needs of children are so great in proportion to the size of their digestive tracts that it becomes important to:

A. avoid liquids until after meals.
B. serve only highly concentrated foods.
C. provide vitamin supplements.
D. serve snacks in addition to meals.

C 22. During the first year of life, the infant increases in length by _______ over what it was at birth.

A. 20%
B. 33%
C. 50%
D. 100%

D 23. The nutrient most often low in the diets of young children in the United States is:

A. vitamin A.
B. protein.
C. vitamin C.
D. iron.

A 24. The food intake of preschoolers is often highly variable because:

A. rates of growth vary.
B. milk is often under-consumed.
C. children are poor judges of their own appetite.
D. children watch too much television.

C 25. Symptoms of the classic allergy response include all the following except:

A. itching.
B. reddening skin.
C. vomiting.
D. asthma.

Chapter 16
Nutrition During Adulthood

I. Points to consider

Chapter 16 is designed to allow you to:

1. Discuss the causes of the principal nutrition problems of adults.
2. List biological changes that occur during the aging process, and discuss how these changes affect nutrient needs of the elderly.
3. Identify several hypotheses on the causes of aging.
4. Make recommendations for dietary changes in the prevention and treatment of nutritional problems in the elderly.
5. List several nutritional programs that are available to help meet nutritional needs of the elderly.
6. Define Alzheimer's disease and outline its progression and relationship to nutritional status of the elderly.
7. Characterize the effects of alcohol on the health and nutritional status of an individual.

II. Word parts

Complete the following exercise using words in Chapter 16.

Word part	Meaning	Examples
ger	old age	________________
morbid	sickness	________________
mort	death	________________
auto	self	________________
chron	time	________________
ostomy	form an opening	________________

III. Flash cards

Cut out and review the flash cards for this chapter in Appendix A.

IV. **Review and synthesis**

A. "In general, American adults both young and old are trying to follow many of the diet recommendations outlined [in the Dietary Guidelines]." Summarize three changes adults have made to improve their diet. Then suggest some changes that still should be made. (575)

Positive changes	Needed changes
a.	a.
b.	b.
c.	c.

B. 1. "This is the first time in history our society will need to deal with such a large population of older people." "The 'graying' of America poses some problems." What are the implications of the above quote? (579)

2. "Life expectancy is the time an average person born in specific year, such as 1996, can expect to live." How has the life expectancy changed in the United States over the last 80 years? (578)

3. "One view of aging describes it as a process of slow cell death beginning soon after fertilization." Summarize how aging is related to a loss in organ reserve capacity. (580)

C. "Although the causes of aging remain a mystery, many hypotheses have been promoted to explain it." Briefly describe three theories of the cause of aging. (581)

a.

b.

c.

D. "Older adults vary more in health status among themselves than do persons in any other age group. This means that chronological age is not so useful in predicting physical health status (physiological age)." Give two examples of how each of the physiological changes below can affect nutritional status and overall health of the elderly. (583)

a. Decreased filtration rate by the kidneys

b. Decreased production of digestive enzymes and acid

c. Decreased motility of the digestive tract

d. Loss of teeth

e. Decreased sense of taste and smell

f. Reduction in muscle tissue

g. Reduction in sense of thirst

E. 1. "Medications and old age often go together." List three common drug-related interactions seen in the elderly. (590)

a.

b.

c.

2. "About 15% of older adults experience significant depression." Suggest three ways depression could affect the nutritional status in the elderly. (593)

a.

b.

c.

F. "To predict the nutritional problems of an older person, it is necessary to know the extent of physiological change caused by aging and whether the person shows early warning signs for long-term poor nutrition."

1. List four nutrition-related diseases that occur more often in elderly adults than in other age groups. Add a dietary recommendation to help compensate for each. (583)

   a.

   b.

   c.

   d.

2. Why is a diet with a high nutrient density recommended for the elderly?

G. "If a 1600 to 1800 kcal diet plan represents too much food energy, a special attempt should be made to regularly choose nutrient-rich foods, such as 1% and nonfat milk, leafy vegetables, fish and lean meat, along with some nutrient-fortified foods, like ready-to-eat breakfast cereals and calcium-fortified orange juice." List five general guidelines for promoting healthful eating in later years. (595)

a.

b.

c.

d.

e.

H. "Nutrition programs for those age 60 and over offer congregate meal programs, which provide lunch at a central location and home-delivered meals (often known as Meals-on-Wheels if sponsored by the local private or public agencies)." The U.S. government sets specific standards for home-served meals and for those served in congregate feeding centers. List two of these meal standards. (597)

a.

b.

V. Applying nutrition to your life

"Overall, good nutrition benefits older adults in many ways. It delays the onset of some diseases; improves management of some existing diseases; hastens recovery from many illnesses; can increase mental, physical, and social well-being; and often decreases the need for and length of hospitalization." (596) Take a look at how eating quick service food can affect adult nutrition. Using the information in Appendix A in your textbook or your NutriTrac software, answer the following questions.

1. If your diet allows you to eat between 500 and 650 kcal of hamburger on a bun, which of the following would be the most nutritious choice?

   a. McDonald's Big Mac hamburger
   b. Burger King's Whopper sandwich

   Why did you choose the one you did? On which nutrients did you base your decision?

2. Perform an analysis of the following choices from a quick service restaurant diet for someone 30 years older than you but of your weight, height, and gender. Compare the vitamin A, vitamin B-6, folate, vitamin C, iron, calcium, zinc, and energy content to the RDA for elderly persons.

   <u>Breakfast</u>

   4 ounces orange juice
   2 Egg McMuffins
   2 cups black coffee

   <u>Lunch</u>

   1 Burger King Whopper
   1 small order of french fries
   12 ounces regular cola drink

   <u>Dinner</u>

   1 Arby's regular roast beef sandwich
   1 small order of french fries
   1 cup black coffee
   1 Dairy Queen banana split

Can you suggest four simple changes to improve this diet?

a.

b.

c.

d.

VI. Chapter 16 summary

Fill in the blanks using the words listed at the end of this summary.

A goal for all of us should be to delay symptoms of and disabilities from ___________ diseases for as many years as possible. Good nutritional habits -- especially following the Food Guide Pyramid and __________________ -- play a role in this process. A basic plan for health promotion and disease prevention includes eating a proper diet, performing regular physical activity, abstaining from smoking, obtaining adequate sleep and fluid, limiting alcohol intake, and limiting stress.

The Dietary Guidelines for Americans recommend that individuals eat a variety of foods; maintain or improve ___________; choose a diet with plenty of vegetables, fruits, and grains; choose a diet low in fat, ___________, and cholesterol; and choose a diet moderate in salt and ___________. For those who drink alcoholic beverages, it is recommended that they do so in moderation.

Although life span has not changed, life ___________ has increased dramatically over the past century. For many societies, this means an increasing proportion of the population is over ___________ years of age. Aging begins before birth. Cell aging results from automatic cellular changes and ___________ influences, such as DNA damage, damage caused by electron-seeking free-radical compounds, _________ changes, high blood _______, and alterations in the _______ system.

Nutritional problems of older adults are related to the presence of chronic diseases and the normal decreases in ___________ function that occur with time. These include loss of teeth, lessened sensitivity of the senses of ___________ and smell, changes in gastrointestinal tract function, and deterioration in heart and ___________ health. Although disease affects nutritional state, the reverse is also true. Immune function is adversely affected by ___________, setting the stage for infection.

___________ disease is a progressive and irreversible brain disorder. The causes are under investigation. It differs from other types of senile dementia in that the brain tissue accumulates abnormal ___________ plaques and tangled nerves. Nutritional health for people in advanced stages of this disease is often complicated by special ___________ problems.

Scientists are only now beginning extensive study of specific nutrient needs of older people. Diet plans should be based on a nutrient-dense approach and individualized for existing health problems, decreased ____________________, the presence of drug-nutrient interactions, possible depression, and economic constraints. Specific nutrients such as protein, vitamin D, _____, vitamin B-6, vitamin B-12, ______________, and zinc -- along with ______ -- often deserve special attention in diet planning.

____________ is an issue for all adults -- from early adulthood through elderly years. Its ability to influence ____________ health is enormous. In the short run, alcohol affects the ___________ more than any other organ. Acting as a sedative, it tends to relieve the drinker's _______________, slur speech, reduce coordination in walking, and impair judgement. Drinking alcohol excessively contributes to certain forms of cancer, cirrhosis of the ___________, motor vehicle and other accidents, suicides, and homicides. __________ drinking for adults is condoned if it can be controlled.

Use the following words to complete the summary:

alcohol
Alzheimer's
anxiety
bone
brain
calcium
chronic
dietary fiber
Dietary Guidelines
environmental

expectancy
feeding
folate
glucose
hormonal
immune
liver
moderate
nutritional

physical abilities
protein
saturated fat
sugar
taste
undernutrition
weight
65

Check your answers using the summary for Chapter 16 in your textbook; use the next page of this <u>Study Guide</u> for the last six answers.

Answers to selected questions

VI. alcohol; nutritional; brain; anxiety; liver; moderate

VII. Practice examination

Cover the answers on your initial attempt.

__A__ 1. Experiments on animals show that the animals who lived the longest were:

A. fed nutritionally balanced diets that contained less energy than the amounts normally eaten by the animal.
B. fed the amounts normally eaten by the animal, but the supply of each specific nutrient was carefully controlled to ensure it always met the RDA.
C. fed nutritious diets in larger amounts than normally consumed by the animal.
D. allowed to eat as much as they wanted at any time they wanted.

__D__ 2. The reason the incidence of obesity increases with age is that:

A. the basal metabolic rate decreases with age.
B. physical activity often decreases with age.
C. energy intake exceeds energy expenditure.
D. all of the above.

__B__ 3. The deficiency of which of the following nutrients may result in anemia?

A. phosphorus, iron, protein, or selenium
B. iron, folate, vitamin B-6, or vitamin B-12
C. calcium, magnesium, folate, or iron
D. vitamin C, protein, iron, or manganese

__C__ 4. To maintain optimal nutritional status and healthy weight, the diet of an elderly person should have a _________ nutrient density and be _________ in energy content.

A. low, high
B. low, low
C. high, moderate
D. high, high

__C__ 5. During aging, the needs for vitamins and minerals;

A. continually fluctuate.
B. greatly decrease.
C. somewhat increase in some cases.
D. greatly increase.

__A__ 6. Hypotheses on aging include all <u>except</u> which of the following ideas?

A. reduced physical activity spares physiological deterioration.
B. cell loss is genetically programmed.
C. partial misdirection of the immune system occurs.
D. intracellular sludge accumulates.

A 7. During mid-life, the most important component of the diet to adjust is:

A. energy intake.
B. water intake.
C. carbohydrate intake.
D. vitamin intake.

A 8. Some ways to reduce the risk of coronary heart disease are:

A. quit smoking and reduce saturated fat intake.
B. reduce exercise to prevent stress on the heart.
C. obtain 50% of total energy intake from fat and decrease carbohydrate intake.
D. all of the above.

D 9. Which of the following does NOT describe a physiological change of aging?

A. decreases in digestion and absorption capacity
B. reduction in lean body mass
C. lower basal metabolism
D. increase in taste sensitivity

C 10. The two key terms for adequate adult nutrition are:

A. varied and minimum amounts.
B. colorful foods and abundance.
C. varied and moderate amounts.
D. similar and adequate.

A 11. Recommendations for preventing osteoporosis include:

A. consuming adequate amounts of calcium from infancy throughout adulthood.
B. consuming more potassium and selenium.
C. increasing the intake of iron, magnesium, and zinc during adulthood.
D. A and B.

C 12. Of the following, the principal nutrition problem of young and middle-aged adults is:

A. anemia.
B. goiter.
C. obesity.
D. hypoglycemia.

D 13. The maximum life span for humans is about:

A. 60 years.
B. 65 years.
C. 85 years.
D. 120 years.

C 14. Common nutrition-related chronic diseases of adults include:

A. asthma, diabetes, and hypertension.
B. hypertension, cancer, and arthritis.
C. atherosclerosis, high blood pressure, and obesity.
D. atherosclerosis, high blood pressure, and kidney disease.

A 15. Some nutrient needs in adulthood are lowered because of decreased needs for:

A. growth.
B. maintenance.
C. physical activity.
D. regulation of body processes.

B 16. To combat the high incidence of overweight and obesity in the United States, many people are reducing their intake of:

A. whole-grain cereals.
B. total energy intake.
C. cholesterol.
D. sodium.

A 17. Americans have reduced intakes of cholesterol and saturated fat in the past few years to decrease the risk of:

A. heart disease.
B. colon cancer.
C. anemia.
D. osteoporosis.

D 18. Because of the high incidence of high blood pressure in the United States, many people are encouraged to lower their intake of:

A. meats.
B. sugars and sweets.
C. dairy products.
D. sodium.

C 19. To help prevent colon cancer, Americans today are increasing their intake of:

A. fresh fruit.
B. lean, red meat.
C. whole-grain products.
D. dairy fats.

B 20. During adulthood, the component of the diet that most often needs reexamination is:

A. water intake.
B. energy intake.
C. carbohydrate intake.
D. vitamin intake.

D 21. At the turn of the century the most common cause of death was:

A. cancer.
B. heart disease.
C. accidents.
D. infectious diseases.

D 22. Nutrition programs such as congregate meals or home-delivered meals provide which of the following?

A. an improved nutritional status
B. a social atmosphere
C. an economical meal for low income elderly
D. all of the above

B 23. Drinking out of aluminum cans causes Alzheimer's Disease.

A. True
B. False

D 24. Among the older populations of the United States, the fastest growing segment of the population is ages:

A. 60 to 65
B. 65 to 70
C. 70 to 80
D. 85+

D 25. The fluid recommendation for the elderly is the same as for younger adults:

A. about 1 milliliter per kcal of energy metabolized.
B. about 2 liters a day.
C. about 8 cups of fluid daily
D. either a, b, or c.

Chapter 17
Food Safety

I. Points to consider

Chapter 17 is designed to allow you to:

1. List some of the types of microorganisms, viruses, and parasites found in food and their general characteristics.
2. Describe the procedures that can be used to control microbial growth in foods.
3. Outline the major types of food-borne illness caused by microorganisms.
4. Compare and contrast food preservation methods.
5. Describe the main reasons for using chemical additives in foods, the general classes of additives, and the functions of each class.
6. List the major categories of common food additives and foods in which they are used.
7. Differentiate between food additives as intentional or unintentional, and describe the importance of the Generally Recognized As Safe (GRAS) list and the Delaney clause.

II. Word parts

Complete the following exercise using words in Chapter 17.

Word part	Meaning	Examples
ferment	leaven	______________
cocci	berry shape	______________
septic	due to decomposition	______________
micro	small	______________
sequester	separate from the whole	______________
botul(us)	sausage	______________

III. Flash cards

Cut out and review the flash cards for this chapter in Appendix A.

IV. **Review and synthesis**

A. "Today scientists know that food-borne illness is caused by specific toxin-producing bacteria and other microbes. These organisms cause health problems either directly by invading the intestinal wall and producing an infection or indirectly by producing a toxin in the food that later harms us (called an intoxication)."

1. List 4 factors that are responsible for food spoilage. (618)

   a.

   b.

   c.

   d.

2. Using the thermometer, indicate: (619)

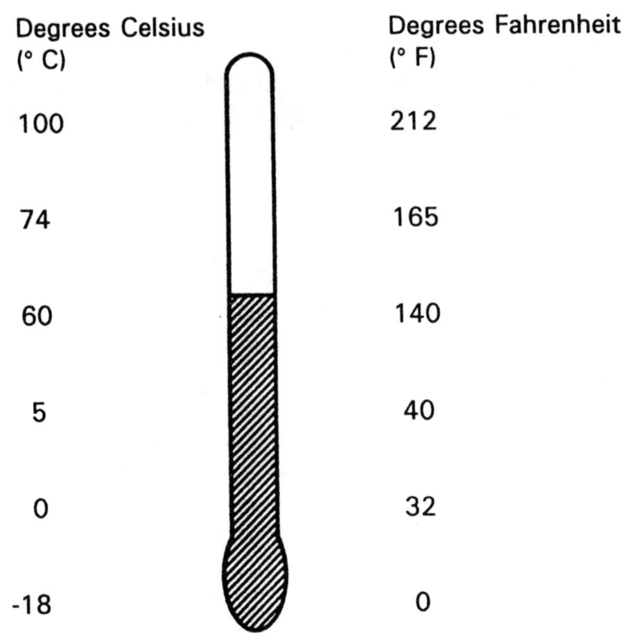

   a. refrigerator temperature

   b. danger zone: where bacteria grow

   c. minimum temperature to cook beef

   d. minimum temperature to cook pork

   e. temperature at which water freezes

   f. temperature range for microbes that likely cause food-borne illness

B. "Every decade the list of microorganisms suspected of causing food-borne illness lengthens." (614)

1. What is the cause of most food-borne illness?

2. What are some other possible causes of food-borne illness?

   a.

   b.

   c.

3. List six general guidelines to follow to avoid food-borne illness. (618)

   a.

   b.

   c.

   d.

   e.

   f.

4. For the following organisms and agents that cause food-borne illness, list their source, symptoms, and specific prevention measures. (615)

	Source	Symptoms	Specific prevention measures
Staphylococcus aureus			
Salmonella			
Clostridium perfringens			
Clostridium botulinum			

C. 1. "In 1958, all food additives used in the United States and considered safe at that time were put on a Generally Recognized As Safe (GRAS) list." Briefly define the GRAS list in terms of its development and use. (627)

2. "If an additive is shown to cause cancer, even though only in very high doses, no margin of safety is allowed. The food additive cannot be used, because it would violate the Delaney Clause in the 1958 Food Additive Amendments." What arguments could you use to support and to question the use of the Delaney clause? (628)

For

Against

D. "Most additives are used to limit food spoilage. Food additives such as potassium sorbate are used to maintain the safety and acceptability of foods by retarding the growth of problem microbes implicated in food-borne illness." (626)

1. Additives are used in food processing for four major purposes. Match each type of additive below to the major purpose.

Additive		Purpose
a. ______	antioxidants	A. increase nutritive value
b. ______	colors	B. preserve freshness
c. ______	emulsifiers	C. aid in processing
d. ______	thiamin and riboflavin	D. improve flavor or appearance
e. ______	flavor enhancers	
f. ______	antimicrobial agents	
g. ______	stabilizers, thickeners, texturizers	

2. Match some common examples of additives to one of the purposes above.

a. ____ nitrates/nitrites	e. ____ monosodium glutamate (MSG)
b. ____ calcium propionate	f. ____ BHA/BHT
c. ____ potassium iodide	g. ____ sulfur dioxide
d. ____ calcium	h. ____ monoglycerides, diglycerides

See page 198 of this Study Guide to check your answers to Part 1 and Part 2.

E. "The question should not be whether a food additive -- such as salt -- is a chemical but rather whether the chemical additive is safe to use." (627) Using Appendix N in your textbook as needed, decipher the role of each ingredient in this food label.

> INGREDIENTS: ENRICHED FLOUR, (BLEACHED WHEAT FLOUR, NIACIN, IRON, THIAMIN MONONITRATE, AND RIBOFLAVIN), VEGETABLE SHORTENING (CONTAINS ONE OR BOTH OF THE FOLLOWING PARTIALLY HYDROGENATED OILS: SOYBEAN, COTTONSEED), SODIUM ALUMINUM PHOSPHATE, MONOCALCIUM PHOSPHATE MONO- AND DIGLYCERIDES, WHEY, SALT, DRIED BUTTERMILK.

Does it make you feel more comfortable to understand <u>what actually</u> is in your food?

F. "Farmers know potatoes must be stored in the dark so that solanine won't be synthesized." Name two natural toxicants that occur in foods and briefly describe their toxic effects. (633)

a.

b.

G. "The presence of mercury in swordfish or shark may concern you, but it's normally not a health risk unless your diet is dominated by these fish." List five environmental contaminants in food, where they are most likely to be found, and a way to reduce each risk. (636)

a.

b.

c.

d.

e.

V. Applying nutrition to your life

"Microbes that cause food-borne illness typically enter food through cross-contamination (usually from improper food handling) and grow because they are maintained at temperatures favorable to them." Assess the potential for food-borne illness where you live. Can you find poor practices in: (612)

a. grocery-shopping habits

b. length of refrigerator storage

c. improper cleaning of the kitchen cutting board after contact with raw meats

d. food preparation

e. extent of cooking

f. attention to leftovers

VI. Chapter 17 summary

Fill in the blanks using the words listed at the end of this summary.

_________ and other microbes in foods are the agents most likely to cause food-borne illness. To guard against food-borne illness in the past, ______, sugar, ______, fermentation, and drying were used. Today, careful cooking, ______, and keeping ______ foods hot and ______ foods cold provide additional insurance. Major causes of food-borne illness today are the bacteria Salmonella, ___________, and ___________. To protect against these microbes, cover ______, do not sneeze on foods, avoid contact between ___________ and other food products, and rapidly _______ and later thoroughly ______ leftovers. Thorough _________ and the use of ________ dairy products further protects against other bacteria and _________. _________ is a common cause of food-borne illness. It occurs when bacteria on raw animal products come in contact with foods that can support bacterial growth. Because of this risk, no perishable food should be kept at ________ for more than ________ hours, especially if a possibility exists that it has come in contact with raw animal products.

Treatment for food-borne illness usually requires ________ extra ________, avoiding touching food while diarrhea is present, thorough _______, and bed rest.

Food additives are primarily used to extend shelf life by preventing microbial growth and destruction of food components by _________, metals, and other substances. Food additives are classified as those ________ added to foods and those that ________ end up in foods. Use of a food additive generally is limited to no more than ______ of the greatest amount that causes no observable symptoms in animals. In most cases the ______ bans use of any intentional food additive if it causes cancer.

Antioxidants, such as _______ and sulfites, prevent oxygen and enzyme destruction of food products. _______ suspend fat in ___________, improving the uniformity, smoothness, and body of foods such as ice cream. Common preservatives include _________ and sorbic acid, which prevent bacterial ______. ___________ bind metals, preventing them from spoiling foods. Toxic substances occur naturally in a variety of foods, such as green potatoes, _______, and _______. Cooking foods limits their toxic effects. Environmental contaminants also can be found in food. Because most of them are ______, trim fat from meats and discard fat that is rendered during the cooking of meats, fish, and poultry. In addition, ______ fruits and vegetables thoroughly.

Most concern about pesticide residues in foods focuses on __________ rather than acute toxicity, since the amounts of residues are extremely __________. Growing evidence, including the problems of contamination of underground ____________, indicates that we would be better off if we ___________ our use of pesticides. Pesticide use in general substantially contributes to the ____________ applied intentionally to the earth's surface. Once a pesticide is applied, it can turn up in a number of __________ places. The primary reason for using pesticides is _______________.

Use the following words to complete the summary:

bacteria
chemical load
chronic
Clostridium perfringens
cold
cooking of foods
cool
cross-contamination
cuts on hands
Delaney Clause
drinking
economic
emulsifiers
fat-soluble
fluids
growth
hand washing
hot
incidentally
intentionally
mushrooms
oxygen
pasteurization
pasteurized
raw fish
raw meat and poultry products
reduced
reheat
room temperature
salt
sequestrants
small
smoke
sodium benzoate
Staphylococcus aureus
unintended
viruses
vitamin E
wash
water
water supplies
1 to 2
1/100

Check your answers using the summary for Chapter 17 in your textbook; use the next page of this Study Guide for the last seven answers.

Answers to selected questions

IV. D. 1. b, d, c, a, d, b, c

2. b, b, a, a, d, b, b or d, c

VI. chronic; small; water supplies; reduced; chemical load; unintended; economic

VII. Practice examination

Cover the answers on your initial attempt.

D 1. Food additives may be used to:

A. destroy nutrients.
B. disguise faulty products.
C. deceive customers.
D. enhance appearance.

B 2. Food additives widely used for many years without apparent ill effects are on the _______ list.

A. FDA
B. GRAS
C. additive safety
D. Delaney

A 3. Vitamin C, vitamin E, and BHA are all:

A. antioxidants.
B. flavor enhancers.
C. antimicrobial agents.
D. incidental food additives.

D 4. It is unwise to thaw meats or poultry:

A. in a microwave oven.
B. in the refrigerator.
C. under cool running water.
D. at room temperature.

A 5. Salmonella bacteria are usually spread via:

A. raw meats, poultry, and eggs.
B. pickled vegetables.
C. home-canned vegetables.
D. raw vegetables.

A 6. Pasteurization involves the:

A. exposure of food to high temperatures for short periods to destroy harmful microorganisms.
B. exposure of food to heat to inactivate enzymes that cause undesirable effects in foods during storage.
C. the fortification of foods with vitamins A and D.
D. use of irradiation to destroy certain pathogens in foods.

B 7. Which of the following is NOT a function of food additives?

A. emulsification
B. help speed the cooking process
C. preservation
D. enhancement of flavor

A 8. The most common cause of food-borne illness is the presence of what in foods?

A. bacteria
B. chemical preservatives
C. viruses
D. molds

C 9. The Delaney clause states:

A. there is a threshold for carcinogens.
B. the Generally Recognized As Safe (GRAS) list must be reviewed every 5 years.
C. no substance either introduced or reevaluated after 1958 that is shown to be carcinogenic can be knowingly added to food.
D. additives must be evaluated for safety.

A 10. The factor that is least important to control in order to limit food-borne illness is:

A. ptomaine synthesis.
B. presence of microbes.
C. temperature of food.
D. time of incubation.

D 11. Indirect additives include:

A. oils and fats in the forms of shortenings.
B. substances that provide a major energy contribution to the food, such as sugar.
C. substances often used at home, such as vanilla and garlic.
D. minerals from cooking vessels.

D 12. Ancient methods of food preservation include:

A. pasteurizing and sterilizing.
B. canning, blanching, and irradiating.
C. freezing and boiling.
D. drying, smoking, and fermenting.

C 13. Regulation of food additives is the responsibility of the:

A. American Medical Association.
B. Department of Agriculture.
C. Food and Drug Administration.
D. National Research Council.

A 14. Aflatoxins:

A. are linked to cancer in animals.
B. are intentional food additives.
C. occur only in corn and peanut products.
D. are on the GRAS list.

B 15. Solanine is:

A. not known to be harmful to humans.
B. a naturally occurring toxin found in green potatoes.
C. a naturally occurring toxin found in shellfish.
D. a toxin that grows on corn and peanut products.

A 16. Substances used to preserve foods by lowering the pH are:

A. vinegar and citric acid.
B. smoke and irradiation.
C. baking powder and soda.
D. salt and sugar.

D 17. In foods, additives known as anticaking agents:

A. incorporate fat into water-based mediums.
B. speed up the process of aging in flour.
C. serve as a flavor enhancers.
D. absorb moisture to keep a product free-flowing.

B 18. Food can be kept for long periods of time by adding salt or sugar because these substances:

A. make the food too acidic for spoilage to occur.
B. bind to water, thereby making it unavailable to microbes.
C. kill microorganisms.
D. dissolve the cell walls in plant foods.

B 19. A danger of using home-canned food if the processing has been inadequate is:

A. cancer.
B. botulism.
C. excessive nutrient loss.
D. excessive tin in the juice.

D 20. Which of the following does not contribute to harmful bacterial growth in foods?

A. exposure to raw poultry or meat juices
B. soil contamination in foods
C. temperatures between 40° F and 140° F
D. cooling foods to adequately low temperatures within 1 to 2 hours

A 21. Nitrite prevents the growth of:

A. C. botulinum.
B. C. perfringens.
C. S. aureus.
D. yeasts.

B 22. The organism that causes food-borne illness and is often associated with small cuts and boils is:

A. Aspergillus.
B. Staphylococcus.
C. C. botulinum.
D. Salmonella.

A 23. Bacteria that can grow in the absence of oxygen are called:

A. anaerobes.
B. molds.
C. aerobes.
D. yeasts.

D 24. The organisms used in the process of fermentation:

A. metabolize all the oxygen in food.
B. produce water in the food.
C. utilize all the nutrients in a food.
D. produce products, such as acids, that inhibit the growth of other organisms.

D 25. Keeping food above 140° F (60° C):

A. increases microbial growth.
B. slows chemical deterioration.
C. decreases chemical reactions.
D. reduces the growth of pathogens.

CHAPTER 18
Undernutrition Throughout the World

I. Points to consider

Chapter 18 is designed to allow you to:

1. Define and characterize the terms hunger, malnutrition, and undernutrition.
2. Evaluate the consequences of undernutrition during critical periods in a person's life.
3. Examine undernutrition in America and highlight several programs established to combat this problem.
4. Examine undernutrition in the Third World and evaluate the major obstacles which hinder a solution.
5. Outline some possible solutions to undernutrition in the Third World.
6. Consider how biotechnology may help solve the food shortage/distribution problem.

II. Word parts

Complete the following exercise using words in Chapter 18.

Word part	Meaning	Examples
mal	abnormal	________________
gen	to become or produce	________________
chron	pertaining to time	________________
bio	pertaining to life	________________
under	beneath	________________
geo	pertaining to earth	________________
pestis	plague	________________
sanita	pertaining to health	________________

III. Flash cards

Cut out and review the flash cards for this chapter in Appendix A.

IV. Review and synthesis

A. 1. "Symptoms of chronic hunger can be found not only in the developing world but also among people living at or below the poverty level in America." List four causes of chronic hunger in the United States. (646-647)

List four causes of chronic hunger:

a.

b.

c.

d.

2. What action would contribute to a solution for one of the four causes you listed above?

B. "Undernutrition is the most common form of malnutrition among the poor in both developing and developed countries." Define and distinguish between the terms malnutrition, undernutrition, and protein-energy malnutrition. (648)

C. 1. "Prolonged undernutrition is detrimental to health at all stages of life but is particularly critical during some periods of growth and old age." Give one example of how undernutrition can jeopardize the health of a pregnant woman, an infant, a child, and an elderly person. (650)

<u>pregnant woman:</u>

<u>infant:</u>

<u>child:</u>

<u>elderly person:</u>

2. List two possible reasons that the infant mortality for African Americans is higher than that for U.S. Caucasians.

a.

b.

D. 1. "In the 1950s, it was assumed that all Americans had enough to eat. Nevertheless, occasional reports of undernutrition surfaced, mostly among the chronic poor." In the 1960s, several programs were started in order to reduce malnutrition. Match the following characteristics with the appropriate program. (You can use a letter more than once.) (655)

Food Stamp Program	School Lunch and Breakfast Program	Women, Infants, and Children (WIC) Program
____________	____________	____________
____________	____________	____________

a. Was revitalized by President John F. Kennedy.

b. Is credited for the recent widespread drop in iron-deficiency anemia.

c. Became nationally available in 1975.

d. Provides food vouchers and nutrition education to low-income pregnant and lactating women and their young children.

e. Stamps are used to purchase food.

f. Enables low-income grade school students to receive meals at reduced or no cost.

E. 1. "Programs which have proven immensely helpful in the United States are only a starting point in this context." List four major obstacles Third World countries must face when dealing with undernutrition. Describe each in one sentence. (660)

a.

b.

c.

d.

2. Discuss how war and civil unrest specifically contribute to undernutrition. (665)

F. 1. "For the most part the solution lies in helping people to meet their own needs and directing them to resources and employment opportunities rather than simply giving them resources." Discuss one of these two solutions for undernutrition in the developing world and indicate why you feel the solution would work. (674)

2. How might biotechnology help reduce undernutrition in the developing world? (680)

V. Applying nutrition to your life

"Overall, life is not necessarily fair, but civilization should try to make it fairer." It is hard not to become distressed over the lack of change in the current world food problem. This chapter has likely made you aware of several problems related to undernutrition in the United States and developing countries. This week, make some contribution to society in order to help solve the problem of undernutrition. In other words, make some attempt to make a difference. Describe your activity below and then act on it.

VI. Chapter 18 summary

Fill in the blanks using the words listed at the end of this summary.

________ is a common thread wherever people suffer from undernutrition. Malnutrition can occur when the food supply is either ________ or abundant. The resulting deficiency conditions or degenerative diseases are influenced by ________ makeup.

Undernutrition is the most common form of ________ in developing countries. It results from inadequate intake, ________, or use of nutrients or food energy. Many deficiency conditions then appear and infectious diseases thrive because the ________ system cannot function properly.

The greatest risk of undernutrition occurs during critical periods of ________ and development: pregnancy, infancy, and ________. Low birth weight is a leading cause of infant ________ worldwide. Many developmental problems are caused by nutritional deprivation during critical periods of ________ growth.

Undernutrition diminishes both ________ and mental capabilities. In poor countries, this is worsened by recurrent infections, ________ conditions, extreme weather, inadequate shelter, and exposure to ________.

In the United States, __________ has been nonexistent since the 1930s, but undernutrition is present. Soup kitchens, food stamps, ______________________, and the Supplemental Feeding Program for Women, Infants, and Children (WIC) have focused on improving the nutritional health of poor and at-risk people. These programs have proven effective in reducing _____________ when adequately funded.

Multiple factors contribute to the problem of undernutrition in developing countries. In densely populated countries, food ________ may be inadequate, as well as means for distributing food may be poor. Farming methods often encourage ________, which deprives the soil of valuable nutrients, thus defeating future efforts to grow food. Limited _______ availability hampers food production. Naturally occurring devastation from droughts, excessive rainfall, ______, crop infestation, and from human causes -- such as urbanization, _________ and civil unrest, debt, and poor sanitation -- all contribute to the major problem of undernutrition.

Proposed solutions to the problem of world undernutrition must consider the interaction of _______ factors, many of which are thoroughly embedded in ________ traditions. Family planning efforts, for example, may not succeed until life ________ increases. Through ______, efforts should be made to improve farming methods, encourage breastfeeding, and improve sanitation and ______. Direct food aid is only a short-term solution. In what may appear to be a step backward, many experts recommend subsistence-level farming, away from the specialization of __________, to increase the economic status of poor people. This is one way to gain meaningful employment and purchasing power for vast numbers of the _______ poor.

"New biotechnology," also known as _______, directly changes some of the genetic material (DNA) of organisms to improve characteristics. It uses a wide range of cell and sub-cell techniques for ______ and then placing genetic material in organisms. It allows access to a wider _______, and it permits faster and more accurate production of new and more useful microbial, ______, and animal species.

Use the following words to complete the summary:

absorption	fire	poverty
brain	gene pool	rain-fed
cash crops	genetic	resources
childhood	genetic engineering	rural
cultural	growth	scarce
deaths	hygiene	school lunch and breakfast program
diseases	immune	synthesizing
education	malnutrition	undernutrition
erosion	multiple	unsanitary
expectancy	physical	war
famine	plant	water

Check your answers using the summary for Chapter 18 in your textbook; use the next page of this <u>Study Guide</u> for the last four answers.

Answers to selected questions

VI. genetic engineering; synthesizing; gene pool; plant

VII. Practice examination

Cover the answers on your initial attempt.

__C__ 1. The largest increase in numbers of chronically hungry people currently occur in:

A. India.
B. The United States.
C. Africa.
D. Asia.

__B__ 2. There are an estimated ________ chronically undernourished people in the world.

A. 75 million
B. 800 million
C. 2.5 billion
D. 7.3 million

__A__ 3. The primary cause of chronic hunger is:

A. poverty.
B. lack of resources.
C. inability to eat.
D. drought.

__D__ 4. The human organism is particularly susceptible to the effects of undernutrition during:

A. pregnancy.
B. infancy.
C. childhood.
D. all of the above.

__C__ 5. Primarily, the consequence of undernutrition both in the United States and worldwide can be seen through a(n):

A. overall decrease in food consumption.
B. decrease in the number of obese people.
C. increase in infant mortality rate.
D. increase in elderly mortality rate.

__C__ 6. Currently there are estimated to be approximately _______ people in the United States living at or near the poverty level.

A. 500 million
B. 30 billion
C. 36 million
D. 100 thousand

__B__ 7. What program has shown to be cost effective in reducing the number of premature, low-birth-weight babies?

A. the Food Stamp Program
B. the WIC Program
C. the School Lunch Program
D. the Congregate Meal Program

__C__ 8. Those at or below the poverty level spend the majority of their money on:

A. insurance.
B. food.
C. rent.
D. alcohol and cigarettes.

B 9. Life expectancy in the United States is approximately ________ times that in developing countries.

A. 1.2
B. 1.5
C. 1.75
D. 2

B 10. In sub-saharan Africa, a woman who is childless is often considered to be:

A. pure.
B. evil.
C. poor.
D. elite.

D 11. In India, bananas may not be fed to children because they supposedly cause:

A. food poisoning.
B. inhibition of growth.
C. nutrient deficiencies.
D. convulsions.

B 12. Which of the following would be considered a delicacy in other countries but would be shunned in the United States?

A. oysters
B. insects
C. brown-shelled eggs
D. pork

D 13. Many of the child deaths each year in developing countries could be prevented if:

A. technology was improved.
B. doctors were more specialized.
C. mothers would learn more about nutrition.
D. sanitation and hygiene were improved.

A 14. In developing countries, there is a growing population shift from:

A. rural to urban centers.
B. urban to rural centers.

C 15. Women in developing countries consider the use of infant formulas as being:

A. expensive.
B. cost-effective.
C. sophisticated.
D. wasteful.

D 16. Human milk is noted for being:

A. hygienic.
B. readily available.
C. nutritionally sound.
D. all of the above.

A 17. The World Health Organization (WHO) estimates that 1.2 billion people are without:

A. a safe and adequate water supply.
B. home and shelter.
C. food.
D. education.

D 18. Developing countries now have two thirds of the world's 19 million people with:

A. cancer.
B. hepatitis.
C. heart disease.
D. HIV infections (AIDS).

A 19. The country that carries the largest national debt is:

A. the United States.
B. Brazil.
C. South Africa.
D. Mexico.

B 20. What hormone produced by cattle has been known to increase milk production when injected into dairy cattle?

A. epinephrine
B. bovine somatotropin (BST)
C. estrogen
D. ADH

D 21. The extreme form of chronic hunger recently seen in Rwanda and Somalia is known as:

A. starvation.
B. malnutrition.
C. undernutrition.
D. famine.

C 22. A barrier to solving undernutrition in the developing world is <u>NOT</u>:

A. external debt.
B. poor infrastructure.
C. a lack of manpower.
D. expanding population.

B 23. A nutrient closely tied to immune function is:

A. calcium.
B. zinc.
C. magnesium.
D. glucose.

C 24. The nutrient most associated with anemia worldwide is:

A. vitamin B-12.
B. copper.
C. iron.
D. vitamin C.

B 25. The U.S. president credited with revitalization of the effort to combat hunger in America is:

A. Eisenhower.
B. Kennedy.
C. Nixon.
D. Reagan.

APPENDIX A

CHAPTER 1

Relate the terms risk factor and chronic disease.

Relate the terms high blood pressure, heart disease, and stroke.

Describe the disease diabetes.

Define the term cancer.

Define the phrase cirrhosis of the liver.

Define the term nutrient.

Define the term metabolism.

What do carbohydrates and glucose have in common?

High blood pressure can injure the arteries that supply blood to the heart and brain. If the injury eventually leads to death of heart tissue, that is part of what is called heart disease. If poor blood flow leads to death of brain tissue, that is referred to as a stroke.

Risk factors are characteristics that make a disease more likely to occur; for example, high blood cholesterol makes heart disease more likely to occur. By definition, a chronic disease takes a long time to develop - chronic means "continuing for a long time."

Cancer refers to the excessive growth of one or more cells in the body, such that they do not respond to normal, physiological controls.

In diabetes insufficient amounts of insulin are produced to keep blood glucose within normal limits. Two forms exist: insulin-dependent, which usually develops in childhood; and non-insulin-dependent, which usually develops in adulthood and is related to excess body fat.

A nutrient is a substance found in food which a human requires in the diet to maintain health.

Cirrhosis refers to substitution of the normal healthy liver cells with connective tissues, usually because a long-standing alcohol intake has poisoned the liver cells.

All carbohydrates are compounds formed from a mixture of carbon, hydrogen, oxygen, and other atoms. Glucose is one example of a carbohydrate.

Metabolism refers to the chemical reactions in the body. These enable cells to release energy from foods, convert one substance to another, and prepare end products for excretion.

Contrast lipids and fats/oils.

Contrast amino acids and protein.

What are vitamins?

Define the term mineral.

Name four nutrition-related diseases that also have genetic links.

Define the term kilocalorie (kcal).

Define the term dietary fiber.

Define the term nutritional status.

Amino acids are the building blocks of protein. Proteins generally are composed of hundreds to thousands of amino acids linked together.

Lipids include compounds that dissolve in ether or benzene. Fats and oils are two such examples. Fats are solid at room temperature, oils are liquid at room temperature - both are classed as lipids.

Minerals are atoms (elements) that both form integral parts of the body structure, such as the calcium in bones, and aid metabolic functions, such as glucose metabolism.

Vitamins are carbon-containing compounds that enable many chemical reactions to occur in the body, some of which unlock the energy-yielding potential of carbohydrates, fats, proteins, and alcohol. Vitamins themselves provide no energy for the body.

A kcalorie (kcal) is the amount of heat it takes to raise the temperature of 1 liter of water 1° C.

- Heart disease
- High blood pressure
- Obesity
- Diabetes
- Cancer
- Osteoporosis

Nutritional status is a measure of the extent to which a person is meeting his or her body's nutrient needs.

Dietary fiber consists of plant substances that are not digested by human enzymes in the intestinal tract. They then contribute to the bulk of the stool.

Based on nutrition surveys, name three nutrients that may be consumed in insufficient amounts in our diets.

Name four important factors that influence our food habits.

What is the approximate percent kcalorie breakdown of the U.S. diet in terms of carbohydrate, fat, and protein?

List the ABCD of nutrition assessment.

Define the word percent.

Represent the prefixes micro, milli, centi, and kilo by numbers.

Illustrate the conversion of a kilogram to pounds, an ounce to grams, a meter to inches, and an inch to centimeters.

A basic plan for health promotion and disease prevention includes which six parts?

Taste, habit, early experiences, routine, one's personal notion of good health, advertising, social factors, and economics

Iron, calcium, vitamin A, and zinc. Dietary fiber is not a nutrient, but it is often poorly consumed as well.

<u>a</u>nthropometric

<u>b</u>iochemical

<u>c</u>linical

<u>d</u>ietary

16% of kcal as protein

50% of kcal as carbohydrates

34% of kcal as fat

micro = 1/1,000,000

milli = 1/1,000

centi = 1/100

kilo = 1,000

The term percent refers to a part of the total when the total represents 100 parts.

- Eat a healthful diet.
- Stay physically active.
- Don't smoke.
- Limit alcohol intake.
- Limit stress.
- Consult health care professionals when necessary.

1 kilogram = 2.2 pounds

1 ounce = 28 grams

1 meter = 39.4 inches

1 inch = 2.54 centimeters

Define the term RDA.

What do these represent?

Define ESADDI.

What is the overall purpose of the Food Guide Pyramid?

If your dietary intake of vitamin C does not meet your RDA, does that mean you necessarily have a poor diet? Why?

Name the six exchange system groups.

What is an "exchange?"

What are phytochemicals?

Why do they deserve our attention?

What is a Nutrition Facts panel?

When must it be used?

ESADDI stands for the Estimated Safe and Adequate Daily Dietary Intake and is set for several nutrients that have no true RDA, including copper, biotin, and chromium.

RDA stands for Recommended Dietary Allowance(s). These are set by the Food and Nutrition Board of the National Academy of Sciences and suggest the amount of a nutrient that should meet the needs of practically all healthy people.

The RDA reflects group - not individual - needs. You may need less than the RDA to maintain health. However, the further you stray from the RDA, the greater your risk for a nutritional deficiency.

The overall purpose of the Food Guide Pyramid is to provide a person with adequate protein, vitamins, and minerals while supplying the bulk of energy from carbohydrate and limiting fat intake.

An "exchange" refers to a proper serving size for a food within an exchange group. For instance, one slice of bread is one starch/bread exchange, as is half a bagel.

Milk group
Fruit group
Vegetables group
Starch/bread group
Meat group
Fat group

A Nutrition Facts panel lists various nutrient quantities in a food, such as energy, protein, carbohydrate, fat, sodium, and vitamins and minerals, compared to the Daily Values. Manufacturers must add a Nutrition Facts panel to almost all foods.

Phytochemicals are constituents in plants that are not nutrients per se but still can provide health benefits. Many phytochemicals are linked to lowering risk for heart disease and certain forms of cancer.

What is a nutrient-dense food?

Contrast the terms:

- positive balance
- negative balance
- equilibrium

The recommendation for energy and sodium intake differ from those for many vitamins.

Relate the terms:

Daily Values (DVs)
Reference Daily Intakes (RDIs)
Daily Reference Values (DRVs)

Define the term essential nutrient.

Name four diseases the Dietary Guidelines are designed to help prevent.

Describe the groups of the Food Guide Pyramid.

What are three suggestions that can improve food choices made from the Food Guide Pyramid?

Positive balance refers to a greater consumption of a nutrient than is excreted, while negative balance is the opposite. In equilibrium consumption equals excretion.

Nutrient density reflects the nutrient content of food in relation to its energy content. Nutrient-dense foods are rich in nutrients compared to energy content.

The Reference Daily Intakes (RDIs) provide estimates for many vitamin and mineral needs. Daily Reference Values (DRVs) provide estimates for carbohydrate, cholesterol, fat, sodium, and dietary fiber needs (or dietary limits). RDIs and DRVs are combined to form the Daily Values.

The RDA for energy is based on average needs. The Food and Nutrition Board warns that the energy RDA is only a rough estimate, and intake should depend on activity. No RDA exists for sodium but there is an estimate of a minimum requirement for health.

The Dietary Guidelines are designed to reduce the risk for chronic diseases, such as heart disease, hypertension, cancer, and cirrhosis of the liver.

An essential nutrient is a nutrient that cannot be manufactured by the body fast enough and must therefore be supplied in the diet.

1) Servings from the milk, yogurt, and cheese group should be low-fat or nonfat.
2) Some servings from beans, nuts, and seeds should be included.
3) Citrus fruits and dark green vegetables should be used.
4) Emphasis should be placed on whole grain breads and cereals.

The Food Guide Pyramid has five groups:

1. milk, yogurt, and cheese
2. meat, poultry, fish, dry beans, eggs, and nuts
3. fruits
4. vegetables
5. breads, cereals, rice, and pasta.

Fats, oils, and sweets are not a group per se.

What is the purpose of the Exchange System?

List the seven Dietary Guidelines.

How are the Daily Values used on the Nutrition Facts panel on a food label?

List the adult servings from the Food Guide Pyramid.

Name two important nutrients found in each food group in the Food Guide Pyramid.

What is one risk associated with the use of health claims on labels?

What does the term "empty calories" mean?

Using protein as an example, describe the term positive balance.

The Guidelines suggest one should 1) eat a variety of foods; 2) maintain or improve your weight; 3) eat plenty of grains, vegetables, and fruit;
4) choose foods low in fat, saturated fat, and cholesterol; 5) choose a diet moderate in sugars; 6) choose a diet moderate in salt; and 7) use alcohol only in moderation, if at all.

The Exchange System arranges foods into 6 different categories designed so that, after noting the proper serving size, each food within a category provides about the same amount of carbohydrate, protein, fat, and energy (kcal).

2 : milk/yogurt/cheese
2-3 : meat/poultry/fish/beans/eggs/nuts
2-3 : fruits
3-5 : vegetables
6-11 : breads/cereals/rice/pasta

moderation : fats/oils/sweets

The Nutrition Facts panel on the label of a food product lists various components of the food as a percentage of their Daily Values. Except for special products, the Daily Values used are for people over 4 years of age.

The whole story may not be told. For example, the benefits from dietary fiber in the food may not be balanced by the problems possible with high intakes.

milk/yogurt/cheese: calcium, riboflavin
meat/poultry/fish/beans: protein, iron
fruits and vegetable groups: vitamins A and C
breads/cereals: thiamin, iron

The fats/oils/sweets category supplies essential fats and vitamin E.

A person in positive protein balance consumes more protein than he or she excretes. This is seen in healthy, growing children and in pregnancy.

A food that supplies energy but offers little nutrient value is often referred to as an empty calorie food.

Define the term quack.

Describe the term organically grown.

Name five beneficial qualities of a food additive.

Why is the term health food so misleading?

Are natural vitamins always superior to synthetic?

Are megadoses of vitamins generally healthful or harmful?

Define herbal therapy.

Define the term epidemiology and provide an example of its use.

Organic growers usually reject pesticides and use natural soil improvers such as compost instead of chemical fertilizers. Also, crop rotation is used to further enrich soil, and biological intervention is used to control pests.

A quack pretends to have medical skills. He or she talks pretentiously without sound knowledge of the subject discussed.

Health food stores often suggest that some foods are "super nutrition foods." However, this is misleading because all foods eaten in moderation are healthy in context of a balanced diet. Likewise, any food eaten in excess can be unhealthy.

Food additives often retard growth of microorganisms, prevent development of off-flavors, keep mixtures from separating, retain food crispiness, and may even raise the nutritional value.

A megadose of a vitamin is defined as an intake of quantities greater than 10 times the RDA. Though bodily chemical imbalances contribute to many diseases, meganutrient therapies have not been accepted as a remedy. Instead, these may cause harmful side effects.

No, the slightly different structure of a few synthetic vitamins do not decrease their value inside the body. Your body usually cannot tell a natural vitamin from a synthetic one. The main difference is the price: "natural" costs more.

Epidemiology is the study of disease patterns in specific populations. For instance, because the classic deficiency symptoms of pellagra appeared in only certain areas of the U.S., it suggested that a specific dietary factor in the diets of those individuals caused the disease.

Herbal therapy uses certain roots, plants, bark, and seeds as medical treatment. Scientific evidence shows that most herbal remedies lack effectiveness and in some cases are dangerous.

Name five ways to spot a quack.

Name two government agencies involved in prosecuting quackery.

Name two appropriate sources of nutrition information.

Contrast hypothesis and theory.

How can freedom of speech and freedom of the press harm the consumer and protect the phoney food promoter?

How do quacks find their victims?

Name four common sources of nutrition quackery.

Describe a double-blind experimental approach.

The Federal Trade Commission is one group who protects persons against false claims. Also, the postal service can act against persons making false claims for products sold through the mail.

Beware when promoters profess that: 1) particular foods can cure specific diseases, 2) only "natural" food should be eaten, 3) modern processing methods strip the nutrition value from foods, 4) sugar is a deadly poison, 5) stress greatly increases your need for nutrients.

A hypothesis is a possible explanation of an event from which to base an experiment. A theory is an idea that is supported by multiple lines of research, or in other words, many hypotheses that have proven true.

Physicians and Registered Dietitians are appropriate sources of nutrition information.

The important aspect of their success is marketing "tender loving care." Clients often praise the people at the health food store because they take time to share "interesting" discoveries in the health field.

Though it would be illegal to label a vitamin as a cure for cancer, if one falsely promotes a product but is not the actual vendor, the person cannot be charged. Retailers often rely on talk shows or magazine articles to provide the misinformation they need to sell store products.

A double-blind experiment tests a hypothesis in a way that neither the subjects nor the researchers know which subjects are receiving the experimental treatment (such as supplemental vitamins) and which subjects are receiving the placebo--"fake"--medicine. The code is broken only after the experiment is over.

1) radio
2) television
3) newspapers
4) books and magazines

Define the term active absorption.

What is required?

CHAPTER 4

What is the life span of a typical absorptive cell?

What does a life span of that magnitude represent in terms of nutrient needs?

Define the term ulcer.

What are two good preventive measures for limiting the risk of developing an ulcer?

What is the key factor that aids absorption of nutrients in the small intestine?

Define the term transit time.

What is a typical transit time?

What is a likely cause of heartburn?

How is the lymphatic system important to nutrition?

Name the bacterium linked to many ulcer cases. What therapy is typically employed in these cases?

The life span of an absorptive cell is about 2 to 5 days. Such a rapid cell turnover puts great demands on the body for nutrients, such as protein, vitamin A, vitamin C, folate, and zinc.

Active absorption is the absorption of a compound from a low concentration into a high concentration. It requires the expenditure of energy and a carrier molecule.

The key factor's are the villi, finger-like projections that extend into the intestine and create a large surface area for absorption.

An ulcer is an erosion of the tissue of the stomach or small intestine. The best way to limit the risk for an ulcer is 1) to not smoke cigarettes, and 2) to not abuse aspirin, alcohol, or other factors that reduce the health of cells of the gastrointestinal tract.

Overeating and especially lying down after overeating are likely causes. A full stomach tends to force food up through the lower esophageal sphincter into the esophagus where the acid chyme irritates the esophagus, causing heartburn.

Transit time refers to the period required for a meal to traverse the gastrointestinal tract. This normally takes 1 to 3 days. There are faster rates in people who consume adequate dietary fiber.

<u>Helicobacter pylori</u>

Therapy induces a combination of antibiotic and antiacid medications.

The lymphatic vessels that serve the small intestine pick up the products of fat absorption and deliver them to the bloodstream. These substances are too large to enter the bloodstream directly.

Indicate the sites of enzyme production in the gastrointestinal tract and its accessory organs.

List and give examples of the increasing biological complexity in the body beginning with cells and ending with an organism.

How efficient are digestion and absorption of food?

What are hemorrhoids and how do they occur?

Describe the role of saliva in digestion.

Describe the major role of the colon.

List the major substances absorbed in the stomach, small intestine, and large intestine (colon).

Describe the function of a sphincter.

Name one sphincter in the gastrointestinal tract.

1.) cells - basic unit of life
2.) tissues - bone, cartilage, muscle, nerve
3.) organs - skin, kidney, liver
4.) organ system - digestive, respiratory system
5.) organism - human body

Enzymes are produced in the mouth, stomach, pancreas, and wall of the small intestine.

Hemorrhoids are swollen veins of the rectum and anus caused by added stress from pregnancy, obesity, prolonged sitting, violent coughing or sneezing, or straining during elimination.

About 90% - 95% of all food substances are digested and absorbed. Little protein, carbohydrate, or fat is excreted in the feces.

The major role of the colon is to finish the absorption of water and minerals from the diet and thus prepare the feces for elimination. Most water and minerals in the diet, however, are absorbed in the small intestine.

Saliva is secreted by glands in the mouth. It contains mucus that envelops and lubricates chewed foods, facilitating passage down the gastrointestinal tract. Saliva also contains enzymes that break down carbohydrates into smaller units.

A sphincter controls flow, acting as a valve.

Pyloric sphincter. This lies between the stomach and small intestine.

stomach - some alcohol
small intestine - peptides and amino acids, monosaccharides (single sugars), monoglycerides and free fatty acids, vitamins, minerals, and water
large intestine - some minerals, water, and fiber by-products

Provide four suggestions for someone who commonly develops constipation.

Name the major parts of the gastrointestinal tract and its related organs.

In what organ does most digestion and absorption occur?

Define the term enzyme and describe the role played in digestion.

Define the term passive absorption. What nutrient is absorbed this way?

In consecutive order, name the parts of the gastrointestinal tract from mouth to anus.

List two ways in which laxatives work. Are they always safe to use?

Define the term villi and describe their function in the small intestine.

The gastrointestinal tract includes the mouth, stomach, small intestine, large intestine, and anus. Entering into the small intestine are the pancreas and the liver (the latter via the gallbladder).

1) Increase intake of food fibers such as bran fiber to draw more water into the intestine thus easing elimination of the stool.
2) Drink adequate water.
3) Eat dried fruits.
4) Perform regular exercise.

Enzymes speed reaction rates. In digestion, enzymes such as pepsin speed the breakdown of food products into the basic components that can be absorbed by the body.

Most digestion and absorption occur in the small intestine, specifically in the duodenum and upper half of the jejunum.

---

mouth

esophagus

stomach

small intestine

large intestine

rectum

anus

Passive absorption is that which requires permeability of the substance through the wall of the small intestine as well as a concentration higher in the small intestine than in the absorptive cells.

Fats are absorbed this way.

Villi are finger-like protrusions in the small intestine. They participate in the digestion and absorption of foodstuffs mostly by increasing surface area of the intestinal tract.

Laxatives work by 1) irritating the intestinal nerve junctions. or
2) drawing water into the intestine to enlarge the stool.

No, with regular use they can decrease muscle action in the large intestine, causing more constipation.

If a person experiences malabsorption of carbohydrate, how will he or she be affected?

Describe those consequences.

Relate sugar intake to dental caries.

Contrast the terms hyperglycemia and hypoglycemia.

What are ketones and how are they linked to a low-carbohydrate diet?

What is the main function of carbohydrate in the body, and for what two types of cells is this function most evident?

Describe why carbohydrates are "protein sparing."

What is phenylketonuria?

In what way is it related to aspartame (NutraSweet)?

Define the term disaccharide and give two examples.

Bacteria on the teeth metabolize sugars into acids that can dissolve the tooth enamel thus leading to dental caries.

Unabsorbed nutrients that make their way into the large intestine stimulate bacterial growth there. This results in the production of acids and gasses, which cause abdominal bloating and discomfort.

Ketones are produced from breakdown products of fatty acids. When insufficient carbohydrate is consumed, fat metabolism is inhibited. The by-products of fat metabolism build up in the liver, which converts them into ketones.

Hyperglycemia means high blood glucose.

Hypoglycemia means low blood glucose.

Cells need glucose for energy production. If you do not eat glucose, the body is forced to synthesize glucose from other nutrients, mainly the amino acids that make up proteins. Carbohydrates in the diet "spare" protein from this use.

Carbohydrate is mainly used for energy production in cells, especially in brain cells and red blood cells. These cells have a limited ability to metabolize other energy-yielding substances.

Disaccharide means double sugar (di- means two). Examples are sucrose -- formed from glucose plus fructose; lactose -- formed from glucose plus galactose; and maltose -- formed from two glucose molecules bonded together.

In phenylketonuria (PKU) a person's liver has a reduced ability to metabolize the amino acid phenylalanine. Since aspartame contains phenylalanine, people with PKU should not use products containing aspartame.

What is the structure of aspartame, and what are two of its characteristics?

Define the term monosaccharide and provide two examples.

Define the term polysaccharide and provide two examples.

Define the term dietary fiber and provide three examples.

Relate the terms fiber and diverticula.

Name the two types of diabetes and their typical causes.

Compare the benefits of soluble and insoluble dietary fibers on the body.

Name two food sources of each.

How much carbohydrate must one eat each day to avoid ketosis?

Monosaccharide means single sugar (mono- stands for one). Examples are glucose, fructose, and galactose.

Aspartame is made of two amino acids and a methanol molecule; therefore it is not a carbohydrate but a protein. It is about 200 times sweeter than sucrose. Aspartame still provides energy (4 kcal per gram) but is so sweet that little is needed.

Dietary fiber refers to foodstuffs that are not digested by human enzymes in the intestinal tract. These include cellulose, hemicellulose, pectins, gums, and mucilages.

Poly--means many, so polysaccharides have many sugar units. Amylose is a straight-chain polysaccharide also called starch.

Glycogen is animal starch and is highly branched.

Insulin-dependent diabetes usually develops in childhood and results from immune system destruction of the insulin-producing cells in the pancreas. Non-insulin-dependent diabetes usually develops in adulthood and is often caused by obesity. Large fat cells are not very sensitive to insulin.

Fiber makes a softer and larger stool which then decreases pressures inside the large intestine during defecation. If a low-fiber diet is consumed, the pressures may be high, causing small pouches called diverticula to pop out in the large intestine wall.

Consuming 50 to 100 grams of carbohydrate a day should prevent ketosis. This amount of carbohydrate should allow for complete fat metabolism.

Soluble dietary fibers found in oats and beans are associated with the lowering of blood glucose and blood cholesterol. Insoluble fibers, found in wheat bran and popcorn, are primarily associated with increased fecal bulk and in turn less constipation.

What are three dietary recommendations for a person who thinks he or she has hypoglycemia?

What are two possible problems from consuming a diet too high in dietary fiber?

Provide some suggestions for a person with lactose intolerance.

Besides reducing the occurrence of diverticulosis, can dietary fiber prevent any other diseases?

What foods do the Dietary Guidelines suggest to encourage an ample carbohydrate intake?

How much dietary fiber should one eat?

Compare the terms soluble and insoluble fiber, especially in terms of their digestibility.

Name three hormones that help regulate blood glucose. Indicate the effect of each.

Very high dietary fiber intakes, such as 60 grams per day, may cause a very large stool that is hard to eliminate and may bind up important minerals, such as calcium, zinc, and iron. In a child's diet the bulkiness of fiber foods may make it difficult to consume enough energy.

A person with hypoglycemia should:

1) consume meals on a regular basis

2) have some protein in each meal

3) have a moderate simple sugar intake

Dietary fiber intake can be used to control blood glucose and blood cholesterol and possibly reduce the risk of colon cancer.

If the person still wants to consume milk products, he, or she can eat smaller portions, yogurt (which supplies its own lactase), cheese (which is naturally low in lactose), and drink milk in which the lactose has already been converted into glucose and galactose.

A reasonable goal is 10 to 13 grams per 1,000 kcal or up to 35 grams of fiber per day.

The Dietary Guidelines suggest increasing the intake of carbohydrates in the form of grains, fruits, and vegetables.

When hyperglycemia develops, insulin attempts to lower blood glucose. When hypoglycemia develops, glucagon, epinephrine, and other hormones break down glycogen in the liver to raise blood glucose.

Insoluble fibers neither dissolve in water nor undergo metabolism by intestinal bacteria. They include cellulose, hemicellulose, and lignins. Soluble fibers either dissolve in water or swell when put into water. They include pectins, gums, and mucilages.

CHAPTER 6

Name the two essential fatty acids.

What are their structures?

Contrast the term lipids with the term fats and oils.

What functions do eicosanoids perform?

What is the current American Heart Association (AHA) recommendation for fat intake?

Contrast omega-3 and omega-6 fatty acids based on their effects on blood clotting.

Name the site where essentially all digestion and absorption of lipids takes place.

What are the five most important risk factors for heart disease?

List three changes a person can make to lower a high blood cholesterol.

Which is the most important change to make?

Lipids include all compounds that dissolve in ether or chloroform.

Fats are lipids that are solid at room temperature, and oils are lipids that are liquid at room temperature.

linoleic acid - 18 carbon atoms, 2 double bonds, omega-6

alpha-linolenic acid - 18 carbon atoms, 3 double bonds, omega-3
The alpha form is the most important nutritionally.

The AHA recommends a diet contain no more than 30% of total kcalories as fat with a ratio of 1:1:1 (10% of kcal each) each of saturated fat, monounsaturated fat, and polyunsaturated fat.

Eicosanoids help control blood clotting and inflammatory responses in the body.

Small intestine

When the body synthesizes eicosanoids from omega-3 fatty acids, there tends to be a decrease in blood clotting and inflammatory processes; eicosanoids from the omega-6 fatty acids generally increase these processes.

1) Reduce saturated fat intake. This is the most important change to make.

2) Reduce cholesterol intake.

3) Increase intake of soluble fiber.

1) Smoking
2) Hypertension (high blood pressure)
3) High blood LDL
4) Diabetes
5) Advancing age

Describe the route that most dietary fats take through the body to arrive at an adipose cell.

What is a phospholipid?

Give an example.

What is the current blood cholesterol cut-off for institution of diet therapy?

Name four functions of fat.

Advertisers tout certain brands of peanut butter as having no cholesterol. Is there something unique about these brands of peanut butter?

Differentiate between the absorption paths followed by long-chain fatty acids versus those taken by short- and medium-chain fatty acids.

What is cholesterol?

How do we obtain cholesterol?

What are two things it does?

Define the term triglyceride.

Where are these found?

A phospholipid is a compound with a triglyceride-like structure but that has only one or two fatty acids. The other sites on the glycerol are bonded to something other than fatty acids; a phosphate group can be part of the additional structure. A common example is lecithin.

Most dietary fats, being long-chained, are absorbed into the intestinal cells and formed into chylomicrons. These travel through the lymphatic system into the bloodstream. The fat is then extracted using the enzyme lipoprotein lipase from the chylomicron and is absorbed into cells.

Fat is used for:

1) energy storage
2) providing energy to the body
3) providing satiety
4) insulating and protecting the body
5) transporting fat-soluble vitamins during absorption from the intestine
6) providing flavor and texture to food
7) forming eicosanoids

200 milligrams cholesterol per 100 milliliters (dl) of serum portion of the blood

Note: dl = deciliter
deci = 1/10 or 10^{-1}

Long-chain fatty acids travel from the small intestine into the lymphatic system; from there they enter the bloodstream.

Short- and medium-chain fatty acids enter directly from the small intestine into the portal vein; from there they travel to the liver.

No, because no plant food has cholesterol. No peanut butter would contain cholesterol if it was free of added animal products.

A triglyceride is a structure with a three-carbon glycerol backbone and three fatty acids attached to the glycerol. Triglycerides are the major form of fat in food and in the body.

Cholesterol is a multi-ringed, waxy substance. Our cells make cholesterol, and we consume it in foods. It is formed into parts of 1) cell membranes, and 2) various hormones and other body structures.

Define the term rancid.

What is nature's natural protection against rancidity?

What is so special about fish oils?

Define the term hydrogenation, and explain why this process is used in foods.

How much fat does one need to consume? Why?

Define the term bile and its role in digestion and absorption.

What are two symptoms of an essential fatty acid deficiency?

Contrast the receptor and the scavenger pathways for LDL uptake.

Define the term emulsifier.

What does it do?

Fish oils contain a high percentage of omega-3 fatty acids, especially EPA and DHA. These compounds tend to reduce blood clotting.

Rancidity reflects the breakdown of polyunsaturated fats at the double bonds. Nature provides vitamin E to protect against the breakdown of the double bonds in a fatty acid and therefore reduce rancidity. In this case, vitamin E acts as an antioxidant.

One needs to consume approximately 1 tablespoon of vegetable oil per day to obtain the omega-6 essential fatty acids. These essential fatty acids are necessary for synthesizing eicosanoids.

Hydrogenation refers to the adding of hydrogen atoms to the carbon-carbon double bonds of fatty acids. This turns liquid oils into solid fats and therefore creates margarines and shortenings that are ideal for making some foods, such as pastries and frostings.

Flaky skin and diarrhea often develop during essential fatty acid deficiency.

Bile, made by the liver and secreted by the gallbladder, breaks large fat globules into tiny droplets. This increases the surface area for enzyme action and ends up speeding fat digestion by enzymes.

An emulsifier, such as bile or lecithin, suspends fat in water, as when lecithin suspends fat in the watery chyme during digestion. In essence, droplets of fat become surrounded by shells of water.

In the receptor pathway, body cells recognize LDL in the bloodstream, take it up, digest it, and use its parts. In the scavenger pathway, white blood cells buried in blood vessels pick up LDL particles and take these up, in turn allowing cholesterol and other fats to invade the blood vessel wall.

Contrast omega-3 and omega-6 fatty acids regarding structure.

What is the "good" cholesterol and the "bad" cholesterol?

Is "bad" cholesterol all bad?

Contrast saturated, monounsaturated, and polyunsaturated fatty acids.

Describe the route of cholesterol synthesized by the liver as it travels from there to cells in the body.

What is an antioxidant?

How does one work?

How does chain length and degree of saturation of fatty acids affect the solid or liquid nature of lipids?

What is a chylomicron?

Define its role in the body.

What is the current recommendation for fish intake?

HDL is the "good" cholesterol because it encourages cholesterol loss from cells. LDL is the "bad" version because it takes cholesterol to cells. However, LDL is only "bad" when it is at high concentrations because it also serves a vital role in the body. Cells need some cholesterol to function.

Omega-3 fatty acids have the first double bond after the third carbon from the methyl ($-CH_3$) end, whereas omega-6 fatty acids have the first double bond after the sixth carbon from the methyl end.

Cholesterol synthesized by the liver is incorporated into a very low density lipoprotein (VLDL). This turns into a low density lipoprotein (LDL) in the bloodstream. Then cells take up the LDL, and by doing so take up the cholesterol initially present in the VLDL.

<u>Saturated</u> fatty acids contain <u>no</u> C=C double bonds in their structure.

<u>Monounsaturated</u> fatty acids contain <u>one</u> C=C double bond.

<u>Polyunsaturated</u> fatty acids contain <u>two or more</u> C=C double bonds.

Long chain length and saturated fatty acids produce solid fats, whereas polyunsaturated fatty acids always produce liquid oils. Note that a short chain length overrides the effects of saturation and produces a liquid oil, even if the fatty acids are saturated, as they are in coconut oil.

An antioxidant is a compound that stops oxidizing agents from taking electrons from compounds. For lipids, antioxidants protect the double bonds present by donating electrons to electron-seeking compounds. Vitamin E is a natural antioxidant.

Eating fish about twice a week is a good dietary practice to obtain omega-3 fatty acids. Note that fish oil supplements are not recommended unless under a physician's guidance.

A chylomicron is a droplet of fat surrounded by a shell of protein and various specialized fats. The chylomicron structure allows fat to travel in the water base of the bloodstream; therefore cells that need the fat have access to it via the bloodstream.

CHAPTER 7

How do proteins specifically contribute to maintaining fluid balance?

How is this linked to edema?

To what does the term complementary proteins refer?

Name four functions of protein in the body.

Describe the "all-or-none" law with regard to amino acid metabolism.

What is the relationship between nitrogen and protein?

Contrast high quality (complete) and low quality (incomplete) proteins.

Name two food sources for each type.

What characteristic does the order of the amino acids give to a protein?

What is the Recommended Dietary Allowance (RDA) of protein for a 154 pound (70 kilogram) man?

When one food protein makes up for the lack of an amino acid in another food protein, the two proteins are said to complement each other; one protein complements the weakness in the other.

Blood proteins counteract the force of blood pressure. As blood pressure tries to force fluid out of the bloodstream, proteins act to attract the fluid back. If insufficient protein is in the bloodstream, excessive fluid leaks out into the tissue spaces; this can lead to edema.

The "all-or-none" law states that if all essential amino acids are not available for synthesizing needed proteins, the amino acids present cannot be used at that time. Thus protein synthesis will not occur.

Proteins 1) produce vital body constituents, such as muscles and blood clotting factors; 2) maintain fluid balance; 3) maintain acid base balance, form hormones and enzymes, contribute to immune function; 4) form glucose when needed; and 5) provide energy for the body.

High quality (complete) proteins contain all nine essential amino acids, whereas low quality (incomplete) proteins lack sufficient amounts of all essential amino acids.

Proteins contain an average of 16% nitrogen. Therefore nitrogen (in grams) times 6.25 = protein (in grams). The same holds if nitrogen is divided by 0.16.

The RDA for protein is 0.8 grams per kilogram of body weight. So 70 x 0.8 = 56 grams of protein.

The order of the amino acids in a protein determines the function of the protein because it dictates its three-dimensional shape.

What does denature represent in terms of a protein?

Define the term amino acid, and contrast essential amino acid with nonessential amino acid.

Describe three types of vegetarianism.

Relate the terms positive, negative, and equilibrium to protein balance.

Contrast kwashiorkor and marasmus.

List the major sites of protein digestion and absorption in the body.

Describe one danger associated with amino acid supplementation.

What is meant by the term limiting amino acid?

An amino acid is a compound with a central carbon atom. Linked to it is an acid group, a hydrogen atom, an amino group, and another chemical group that gives the amino acid its identity. Essential amino acids must be present in the diet. Nonessential amino acids can be made by the body.

If the three-dimensional structure of a protein is destroyed by acid or alkaline solutions, agitation, heat, or other processes, this is called denaturation.

In positive protein balance one would be gaining protein tissue, such as during growth or pregnancy. Negative protein balance refers to a loss of protein tissue, such as occurs during starvation or illness. Protein equilibrium refers to body maintenance, which occurs in adulthood.

Vegans are total vegetarians and eat only plant foods. Fruitarians eat primarily fruits, nuts, honey, and vegetable oils. Both need to ensure some food they eat is fortified with vitamin B-12. Lactovegetarians add dairy products. Lacto-ovo vegetarians add dairy products and eggs.

digestion: stomach
small intestine

absorption: small intestine

Kwashiorkor is a disease that primarily affects young children who are already ill and follow a diet inadequate in energy and especially low in protein. The child develops edema but has fat stores.

Marasmus develops in infants from essentially a starvation diet that is grossly inadequate in both protein and energy. The infant does not show edema and has little or no fat stores.

The essential amino acid in shortest supply in a food or diet limits the amount of protein the body can synthesize.

Amino acid supplements may trigger imbalances in the body which occur because chemically similar amino acids compete for absorption into the blood. An excess of one can create high demand for a carrier and hamper the absorption of another amino acid.

CHAPTER 8

What is the name for the niacin deficiency disease, and what are two of its symptoms?

List two functions of vitamin D.

What is a vitamin?

Can high intakes of water-soluble vitamins be harmful?

If so, which two vitamins are examples?

Provide one example of how vitamins A, D, E, and K are different from the other vitamins?

List two ways water-soluble vitamins are lost in cooking.

Define the term coenzyme.

Name two of the best food sources of riboflavin.

What is our main food source?

Vitamin D helps regulate absorption of calcium and phosphorus and the deposition of calcium in bones.

Pellagra is caused by a prolonged niacin deficiency. Symptoms include the four "D"s - diarrhea, dermatitis, dementia, and death.

When taken in large doses (more than 100 times the RDA), water-soluble vitamins can be toxic, especially vitamin B-6 and niacin.

Vitamins are carbon-containing (organic) compounds needed by the body via diet in small amounts for important metabolic reactions.

Water-soluble vitamins are easily lost in cooking because of heat, alkalinity, and leaching into the cooking water.

Vitamins A, D, E, and K are fat-soluble, whereas the B vitamins and vitamin C dissolve in water.

Liver, mushrooms, spinach, and milk are the most nutrient-dense sources of riboflavin. Milk products are our major food contributors.

Coenzymes are structures that directly help enzymes function.

Name two nutrient-dense sources of niacin and a component in food that can form niacin.

Do nutrition experts recommend general use of a vitamin and mineral supplement?

What is one function of pantothenic acid?

List two good food sources of thiamin.

What is the main function of biotin? Name two sources.

What three B-vitamins participate in homocysteine metabolism?

What is the most important function of vitamin B-6?

What is the term for a thiamin deficiency?

What body functions quickly show signs of it?

No, nutrition experts believe that a diet following the Food Guide Pyramid provides a diet sufficient in vitamins and minerals for most healthy persons.

Mushrooms, wheat bran, tuna and other fish, chicken, asparagus, and peanuts are good sources. Each 60 milligrams of dietary tryptophan remaining after protein synthesis forms 1 milligram of niacin.

Foods containing a very high nutrient density of thiamin are pork products and sunflower seeds. Other good sources include whole grains, green beans, and organ meats.

Pantothenic acid allows many important energy-yielding reactions to take place, such as those in glucose and fat metabolism.

vitamin B-6
folate
vitamin B-12

Biotin acts as a coenzyme in fat and carbohydrate by adding carbon dioxide to other compounds. Sources include cauliflower, egg yolk, cheese, and liver, and it is also produced from intestinal synthesis by bacteria.

Beriberi is the name of the thiamin deficiency disease. Brain and nerve action suffer in a thiamin deficiency.

Protein metabolism is the most important function of vitamin B-6.

Is it necessary to obtain all vitamins daily?

List two functions of vitamin A.

Why are fat-soluble vitamins potentially harmful, and which are especially toxic?

Besides preformed vitamin A, in what other form does vitamin A activity exist in the diet?

Relate the term oncogene to cancer.

Relate a deficiency of vitamin E to a typical result, thc breakdown of red blood cells.

List two good food sources of vitamin D.

Explain the role of the intrinsic factor in vitamin B-12 absorption.

Vitamin A functions to do the following:

1) Maintain vision.

2) Ensure the health of the immune system.

3) Direct aspects of growth and development.

Ideally, vitamins in food should be consumed daily, but an occasional lapse of intake for even the water-soluble vitamins is not harmful.

Potential vitamin A is present as the common plant pigments called carotenes or carotenoids.

The fat-soluble vitamins, especially vitamins A and D, are poorly excreted and thus can easily reach toxic amounts in the body.

A deficiency of vitamin E causes the breakdown (hemolysis) of red blood cells, especially in infancy. Vitamin E protects the polyunsaturated fatty acids and vitamin A in the cell membrane from destruction.

Oncogenes are pieces of genetic material that form blueprints for proteins that can cause cell growth. Chemicals and viruses can alter the oncogenes in humans in such a way that human cells can then grow autonomously. This can lead to cancer.

The intrinsic factor (IF), a protein produced in the stomach, binds to vitamin B-12 in the small intestine. IF is necessary for the adequate absorption of vitamin B-12 in the ileum.

Good food sources of vitamin D include fish oils, fatty fish, and fortified milk.

Name two good food sources of vitamin B-6.

What are the three main functions of vitamin C?

What is the main danger of vitamin B-6 toxicity?

Name three nutrients linked to a reduction in cancer.

How do they act?

What is a key function of folate?

What are two nutrient-dense sources of folate?

Why does a folate deficiency lead to anemia?

Why does FDA limit the amount of folate allowed in a vitamin supplement?

Vitamin C is important for healing wounds, enhancing iron absorption, and acting as an antioxidant.

Meats, fish, and poultry are the best sources, since the vitamin B-6 present in animal foods is better absorbed than that in plant foods.

Nutrients such as beta-carotene, vitamin E, vitamin C, and selenium have potential anticancer properties. They all act as part of antioxidant systems or are antioxidants themselves.

Irreversible nerve damage can result from intake of 2 to 6 grams of vitamin B-6 per day for 2 or more months.

Green leafy vegetables, organ meats, sprouts, and orange juice are the best folate sources.

Folate is necessary for cell division because it contributes to the formation of DNA and RNA.

Excess folate intake can mask the early warning signs of a B-12 deficiency, a potentially dangerous condition necessitating early treatment.

In a folate deficiency, red blood cells can continue to produce enough protein to grow, but they cannot synthesize enough DNA to divide. The resulting large, immature cells lead to a reduction in oxygen-carrying capacity of the blood, in part due to a reduced lifespan of the cells. Thus anemia results.

What is the main function of vitamin K?

Describe how an antioxidant functions.

List three good food sources of vitamin A.

Define xerophthalmia.

At what level of intake is vitamin A considered potentially toxic?

Name two nutrient-dense food sources of vitamin E.

Briefly describe the three stages of the cancer process.

What are three dietary recommendations to reduce the risk of cancer?

An antioxidant such as vitamin E donates electrons to an electron-seeking free radical compound, in turn neutralizing it. This then protects other molecules from attack by the electron-seeking compounds.

Vitamin K is essential for blood clotting because it helps impart a calcium-binding ability to certain blood proteins.

Xerophthalmia, literally "dry eye," is a disease process initiated by a prolonged vitamin A deficiency in which the mucus-forming cells in the eye no longer function properly. Blindness eventually can result.

Foods with the highest nutrient density for vitamin A are carrots, liver, spinach and other greens, sweet potatoes, and yellow squash.

The best sources of vitamin E are plant oils, margarine, and asparagus.

Toxicity symptoms from excessive vitamin A intake are apparent with long-term supplement use at only 5 to 10 times the RDA, especially during pregnancy.

Avoid obesity, reduce fat intake to less than 30% of total energy intake, eat more high fiber foods, eat foods rich in vitamins A and C, avoid excessive amounts of alcohol, and use moderation when consuming smoked or salt-cured foods.

Initiation -- chemicals, radiation, or viruses alter DNA.
promotion -- alcohol, estrogen, and dietary fat encourage division of altered cells.
progression -- the developing cancerous tumor grows and invades surrounding tissues, eventually reaching lymph and blood vessels.

CHAPTER 9

Define the term bioavailability.

What is a potential danger from taking excess mineral supplements?

What two nonmineral substances can affect the bioavailability of minerals?

Name three excellent sources of iron.

What major role does water play in chemical reactions.

Contrast major and trace minerals.

Contrast the absorption rates for heme and nonheme iron.

Contrast the occurrence of iron deficiency and iron-deficiency anemia.

An excess intake of one mineral can influence the absorption and metabolism of other minerals; for example, a high zinc intake reduces copper absorption.

Bioavailability refers to the body's ability to absorb a nutrient from the diet.

Spinach, oysters, liver, clams, peas, and legumes are the most nutrient-dense sources of iron. Beef is also a good source.

Phytic acid in grain fibers and oxalic acid in leafy vegetables both can bind minerals and greatly decrease their absorption.

Major mineral needs are $\geq$ 100 mg per day; trace mineral needs are $<$ 100 mg per day.

Water serves as a medium in which chemical reactions take place. It also actively participates in some chemical reactions.

More people have low iron stores than overt iron-deficiency anemia.

Heme iron is absorbed more efficiently than nonheme iron, about 20% versus 2% to 20%.

Name two groups that are at risk for iron deficiency. Why?

Name two food sources of copper.

What is a function of manganese in the body?

What is the effect on copper status of excessive use of zinc supplements?

What are two food sources of fluoride?

Name and describe a condition that results from prolonged iodide deficiency.

What is the most understood function of chromium?

Name two sources of selenium for a diet.

Copper is primarily found in liver, cocoa, legumes, and whole grains.

Infants, preschoolers, adolescents, menstruating women, and pregnant women are at risk for iron deficiency because their iron needs often exceed their usual iron intake.

Since copper and zinc compete with one another for absorption, overzealous supplementation of zinc can result in a copper deficiency.

Manganese is a component of many different enzymes, such as those used in carbohydrate metabolism, and is important in bone formation.

A goiter develops in an iodide deficiency as the thyroid gland enlarges, attempting to take up more iodide from the bloodstream. The growth failure and mental retardation associated with cretinism occurs in infants whose mothers had iodide-deficient diets during pregnancy.

Tea, seafood, and seaweed are the only good food sources of fluoride. Tap water is a main source, as is toothpaste.

Fish, meats, organ meats, eggs, shellfish, and grains grown in selenium-rich soil are good food sources.

Chromium aids glucose uptake by the cells.

Estimate the fluid needs of an adult.

Name a function of fluoride in the body.

Compare the calcium intake of women over age 25 with their RDA for calcium.

Why is sodium's presence in the diet not necessarily a problem for everyone?

Describe the mechanism that limits iron absorption when iron stores are adequate.

What piece of advice should be given to the general public concerning prevention of high blood pressure?

Name three food sources of phosphorus in the diet.

Name the two good sources of iodide.

During teeth and bone development, fluoride allows for the production of tougher tooth crystals, which are more resistant to acid erosion.

Water needs for an adult can be roughly estimated as 1 milliliter per kcal of energy output.

Only some persons are susceptible to sodium-linked high blood pressure. Even among people with high blood pressure, only part of the condition is caused by an excessive sodium intake.

The RDA for calcium is 800 milligrams, whereas the average calcium intake of women ranges from 500 to 650 milligrams. About 25% of women consume less than 300 mg daily.

To limit the risk of high blood pressure, consume a diet based on the Food Guide Pyramid, rich in whole grains, fruits, and vegetables. This provides ample potassium, calcium, and magnesium and a moderate amount of sodium. In addition, do not become obese, do remain physically active, and don't abuse alcohol.

The blood protein that carries iron is full when iron stores are adequate. This limits transfer of iron absorbed into intestinal cells to the bloodstream. This iron is then likely to be sloughed off with the intestinal cells and excreted.

Saltwater fish, seafood, plants grown near the sea, and iodized salt are the best sources of iodide.

Milk, cheese, bakery products, and meat provide most of the phosphorus in the diet.

Name three functions of magnesium.

How can young women attempt to limit their future risk for osteoporosis?

Name three food sources of magnesium in the diet.

Name two functions of phosphorus.

What are the two major functions of sodium?

Name two major functions of chloride.

Compare the amount of sodium added in food processing with that added during cooking and at mealtimes.

How are copper metabolism and iron metabolism related?

Young women can limit their future risk for osteoporosis by doing the following:

1) Consuming at least the RDA for calcium
2) Performing regular physical activity
3) Maintaining regular menses
4) Avoiding tobacco and moderating alcohol use if applicable

Magnesium is an important cofactor for numerous enzymes. Proper nerve and cardiac functions require magnesium.

Phosphorus is a component of enzymes, ATP, cell membranes, and bone.

Whole grains, broccoli, squash, bran, nuts, and seeds are excellent magnesium sources. Excellent sources are plant products.

Chloride forms a negative ion that is an important part of extracellular fluid. These ions also are part of stomach acid and are used during immune responses.

Sodium is the major positive ion of extracellular fluid and is partly responsible for fluid balance in this and other compartments. Sodium is also important in nerve cell conduction.

A copper-containing protein aids in iron metabolism. Copper deficiency can lead to an iron deficiency.

Approximately one third to one half the sodium in the diet is added in cooking or at the table. One half is a result of manufacturing procedures. Very little occurs naturally in foods.

Name three major functions of zinc in the body.

Name three good food sources of zinc.

Compare the minimum requirement for sodium to our average daily intakes.

Name three major functions of calcium in the body.

Where is most of the potassium found in the body? Name two functions of this mineral.

Compare the composition of healthy bone versus bone in osteoporotic people.

Is this the same difference as seen in rickets and osteomalacia?

Name three good food sources of potassium.

Name three major contributors of calcium in the diet.

Oysters, shellfish, beef, and turkey are rich in zinc. Generally, protein-rich foods are good sources of zinc.

Major functions of zinc include DNA and protein metabolism, wound healing, growth, vitamin A mobilization, proper immune function, and proper development of sexual organs and bones.

Calcium is essential for bone health, blood clotting, muscle contraction, and nerve transmission.

The minimum requirement for sodium is 500 milligrams daily, whereas the average American intake is more than 6 times that, 3 to 7 grams daily. That is equivalent to 7.5 to 18 grams of salt daily.

The bone composition in osteoporosis is essentially the same as normal bone; however, less total bone exists throughout the body.

No, bone in rickets and osteomalacia has decreased calcium content compared with normal bone.

Almost all the potassium in the body is in the intracellular fluid. Its functions are analogous to those of sodium, namely fluid balance and nerve transmission.

Dairy products such as milk and cheese provide most of the calcium in the diet. White bread and rolls also are contributors.

Fruits, vegetables, milk, whole grains, and meats are all good potassium sources.

List three reasons why the body resists weight loss.

Is there any evidence to support the idea that eating meat and potatoes will stop the digestion of both foods?

In addition, should one consume exclusively fresh fruits before noon as some fad diet books suggest?

Why is weight loss generally so rapid in the first week of the diet?

Why should the prevention of obesity be emphasized?

Losing about 1 to 2 pounds of weight per week is typically a goal of sound weight loss plans.

Justify that recommendation for the rate of weight loss.

What is the three-pronged approach that a well-designed diet should take?

What are the best foods to consume when trying to lose weight?

What is the lowest energy consumption per day that still allows for an adequate diet?

Not for any reasons that I can think of.

These ideas are pure nonsense.

1) Thyroid hormone output and therefore basal metabolism drop.
2) The fat storage enzyme can increase activity in the adipose cells.
3) The energy cost of physical activity decreases as body weight decreases.

Prevention of obesity is important because only about 5% of people who diet lose weight and remain that weight. The evidence is strong that people can lose weight, but few can maintain that lower weight.

When dieters cut food intake, they often decrease salt intake. This slightly reduces fluid in the body. If the dieters reduce carbohydrate intake, this reduces glycogen stores in liver and muscles. Both factors contribute to an initial rapid weight loss.

1) Reduce energy consumption.

2) Alter problem behaviors that contribute to overweight and overeating.

3) Increase physical activity.

A pound of fat tissue storage represents about 2700 kcal. Divided by 7 days, the dieter must reduce energy intake by about 400 kcal to lose 1 pound per week or 800 to lose 2 pounds per week. This is the limit of energy reduction to still leave enough energy for obtaining an adequate diet.

Between 1500 and 1800 kcal per day is the lowest recommendation. Below this amount of energy women should consume some vitamin and mineral-fortified foods, such as breakfast cereals, to obtain enough iron.

High-carbohydrate foods are the best foods because carbohydrates provide less than half as many kilocalories as fat. In addition, high-carbohydrate foods are often bulky and therefore lead to a feeling of fullness.

Contrast direct and indirect calorimetry.

About how many kcal are used each day for the thermic effect of food?

Briefly describe the three major categories of energy use by the body.

What physiological factors determine the rate of one's basal metabolism?

How much energy is used for this process?

Provide three suggestions for gaining weight for adults.

Does moderate obesity carry a social stigma it does not deserve based on medical consequences?

List five aspects of a good weight-loss diet.

What five types of behavior modification can help the weight-loss process?

The thermic effect of food represents about 5% to 10% of energy use. Given a 3000 kcal diet and using the 10% figure, this would account for 300 kcal.

Both methods estimate energy use by the body. Direct calorimetry measures the heat the body gives off. Indirect calorimetry measures oxygen consumption (or carbon dioxide output) and estimates the energy use associated with the use of that much oxygen.

One's rate of basal metabolism primarily depends on body surface area and lean body mass. A larger surface area and larger lean body mass yield a higher basal metabolism. A rough estimate is 1 kcal per minute, or 1440 kcal per day.

basal metabolism -- the energy required to keep the resting body alive

thermic effect of food -- the increase in energy use associated with digestion, absorption, and metabolism of energy-yielding nutrients

physical activity -- any energy use for other than the two previous categories

You could argue "yes" in that the social stigma associated with being 20 to 30 pounds overweight is often much greater than the health consequences the extra weight brings.

1) The person could gradually increase consumption of energy-dense foods, such as those higher in fat.

2) Higher-fat foods could be eaten at the end of the meal so that they do not lead to early satiety.

3) Snacks made of dried fruits, bananas, nuts, and granola could be eaten regularly.

1) chain breaking
2) stimulus control
3) cognitive restructuring
4) contingency management
5) self-monitoring

A good weight loss diet will (1) meet nutritional needs, (2) accommodate the dieter's habits and tastes, (3) include a range of readily obtainable foods, (4) promote changing habits that lead to overeating, amd (5) encourage regular physical activity.

Contrast hunger, appetite, and satiety.

How is body mass index calculated?

What is the cutoff value for obesity?

Provide a way to calculate a rough estimate for total energy needs.

What does the term healthy body weight represent?

Briefly describe three ways to determine the amount of body fat in a person.

What body shape is more closely associated with health risks from obesity?

What constitutes a "thrifty" metabolism?

In what ways might it be "thrifty"?

Provide an example of the effect of both nature and nurture on obesity.

Body mass index = weight in kilograms/height^2 in meters; values > than 30 suggest obesity.

A desirable value is approximately 19 to 25.

Hunger is the physiological drive to find and eat food, whereas appetite represents the psychological drive to do so. Satiety should result from fulfilling hunger or appetite impulses because it represents a lack of desire to eat food.

A person of healthy weight shows good health and performs daily activities without weight-related problems. A body mass index of 19 to 25 is one measure of healthy weight, although weight in excess of this value may not lead to ill health. This suggests that healthy weight is best determined in conjunction with a thorough health evaluation by a physician.

Sedentary people need about 9 kcal per pound of body weight. Light activity requires about 13 kcal per pound. Heavy activity requires approximately 20 kcal per pound.

Upper body (apple shape) obesity is more associated with health risks than the lower body (pear shape) obesity. Upper body distribution represents a waist to hip circumference ratio > 0.8 in women and > 1.0 in men.

Body fat can be estimated by the following:

1) measuring skinfold thickness in various sites in the body

2) measuring the resistance of the body to electrical current using a bioelectrical impedance instrument

3) underwater weighing, which is the most accurate but least used method

For nature, identical twins raised apart tend to have similar weight gain patterns.
For nurture, men tend to become obese in middle age, whereas women tend to develop obesity during grade school years.

In the thrifty metabolism concept, some individuals naturally need less energy than others and therefore more easily gain weight and lose weight with more difficulty. A thrifty metabolism could be generated by less fidgeting or by an increased efficiency for synthesizing cellular energy.

When should a very low calorie diet (VLCD) be used to treat obesity?

What does it entail?

What is a "set point".

How powerful is the set point for weight?

Define the term energy balance.

What role does the hypothalamus play in hunger regulation?

What is the basis behind behavior modification?

Simplify the terms stimulus control and contingency management.

What are two tip-offs that suggest a diet is a "fad" diet?

When is gastroplasty used to treat obesity?

What does it entail?

When using physical activity to help lose weight, what is the key factor on which to concentrate?

A "set point" for weight refers to the day-to-day constancy of body weight. Factors tend to keep body weight constant, but statistics show adults increase in body weight over a period of 20 years. Thus the set point is not perfect.

A very low calorie diet (VLCD) could be considered if the person is 40% over healthy body weight and has failed more conventional diet approaches. The VLCD contains 400 to 800 kcal and relatively little carbohydrate.

The hypothalamus has certain centers of cells that probably monitor the levels of energy-yielding nutrients, such as glucose, amino acids, and fatty acids in the bloodstream. A high amount of energy-yielding nutrients leads to satiety; a low amount leads to hunger.

Energy balance is the comparison of energy intake from foods versus energy output, and it also considers changes in energy stores, as in fat stores. If a person's energy intake exceeds energy output, that person will gain weight. If energy intake is less than output, weight will be lost.

Two possible tip-offs are as follows:

1) Quick weight loss is promoted. This is impossible if one is talking about fat loss.

2) There is no attempt to permanently change eating habits. The dieter follows the diet, loses the weight, and then returns to previous eating habits.

The basic approach of behavior modification if to reshape one's environment so that weight maintenance rather than weight gain is the overwhelming thrust. Stimulus control refers to minimizing the factors in one's life that encourage overeating. Contingency management involves setting a plan to deal with diet lapses.

Duration is the key factor rather than intensity. An activity should last long enough to burn 200 or more extra kcal. That requires about 1 hour of brisk walking.

Gastroplasty is used to treat severe (morbid) obesity. (Recall that one measure of severe obesity is when a person is 100 pounds overweight.) Gastroplasty calls for reducing the size of the stomach to approximately the size of a shot glass. This then limits meal size and reduces overeating.

Define metabolism.

Describe anaerobic glycolysis and when it is used.

Give an example of an anabolic pathway.

List one ergogenic aid athletes use in an attempt to raise one's blood concentration of fatty acids. What is the overall purpose of this practice?

Give an example of a catabolic pathway.

Outline the process of carbohydrate loading.

Briefly describe one advantage and one disadvantage of using the splitting of phosphocreatine to form ATP.

Why is it important to distinguish between high carbohydrate versus high fat meals for the athlete?

Anaerobic glycolysis is seen when the oxygen supply is limited or when physical activity is intense. Glucose is broken down into a three-carbon compound that accumulates in the muscles and is converted to lactic acid.

Metabolism is a term that encompasses all chemical processes in the body. In other words, it includes any sequence of chemical processes from beginning to end.

Consuming caffeinated beverages is one practice. This is done in an attempt to utilize more fat during prolonged activity, thereby sparing muscle glycogen stores.

Anabolic pathways build compounds using simple molecules such as O_2, H_2O, and CO_2 in a specific way to form fatty acids, glucose, or even complex cholesterol molecules

Six days before competition, consume 450 grams of carbohydrate per day. During the 72 hours before the event, closer to 600 grams per day is recommended. A gradual decrease in exercise intensity is also recommended in the few days before competition.

Catabolic pathways break down compounds into smaller units; for example, glucose and fatty acids broken down into CO_2 and H_2O.

Fat won't make glycogen, but carbohydrate will.

Advantage: PCr it can be activated instantly.

Disadvantage: There is not enough PCr stored in the muscles to sustain a high rate of ATP resupply for more than a few minutes.

Outline a muscle bulking diet.

Define the term ergogenic aid and give some examples of those that have been supported by scientific evidence.

List three ways iron can be lost in the female athlete.

A physically active lifestyle can reduce many risks of chronic diseases. Provide three examples of those diseases.

Describe a preevent meal.

Give three basic components every exercise program should consist of and the amount of time that should be spent on each.

Describe a postevent meal.

What is the recommended intake of a carbohydrate solution before and during prolonged physical activity? Give the amount and percentage of each.

Ergogenic (work-producing aids) are used to achieve better performance. Those that have documented scientific evidence include sufficient water, lots of carbohydrates, and a balanced diet.

During muscle building, athletes should consume 1.2 to 1.6 grams of protein per kilogram of body weight per day. This is slightly above to twice the RDA of 0.8 grams/kilogram.

- heart disease
- diabetes
- obesity
- high blood pressure

1) sweat loss
2) foot-strike destruction of red blood cells
3) iron loss during menstruation

Warm-up: 5 to 10 minutes

Work-out: 20 or more minutes

Cool-down: 5 to 10 minutes

A preevent meal should include a light meal eaten 2-4 hours before an endurance event to pay glycogen stores. The meal should consist of primarily complex carbohydrates, contain little fat or dietary fiber, and include a moderate amount of protein.

20 to 30 minutes before:	1-2 cups of water or a 10% to 20% CHO solution
During exercise:	1 cup of a 6% CHO solution (like a sports drink) every 15-20 minutes

A postevent meal should contain a large portion of carbohydrate. This should be consumed within 2 hours of the event, and sooner is better. Food such as candy, sugared soft drinks, fruit juice and sports-type carbohydrate supplements can aid in reloading muscles with glycogen right after exercise.

Name the first three steps in the behavior change process.

Quick service foods are characteristically high in ___________

Name the final two steps in the behavior change process.

Is it more effective to attempt to change behavior using small steps or to address the entire behavior change at once?

How can keeping a food diary help in the behavior change process?

Describe the term reinforcement.

Describe how a good behavior change plan evolves.

What four parts should be included in a behavior contract?

Fat

In behavior change, a person must 1) become aware of the problem, 2) study the problem and develop a receptive frame of mind for change, and then 3) attempt a trial change.

Attempting a series of small and perhaps easier changes makes success with the big problem more attainable. The success with each step provides motivation.

One must receive positive reinforcement for the new behavior in order to adopt it successfully into one's lifestyle.

Reinforcement is a reaction by others in response to a person's behavior. Positive reinforcement entails encouragement; negative reinforcement entails criticism or penalty.

A food diary can be an effective tool for gathering baseline information about present behavior. Review of the diary may reveal patterns, associations, and areas that need improvement.

A behavioral contract should include the following:
1) a list of goal behaviors
2) objectives
3) ways to measure progress
4) regular rewards for meeting the terms of the contract

A good plan evolves from rational, deliberate decisions made after considering all options. All information at hand should be incorporated.

What are three primary and three secondary factors that drive our food choices?

List three ways to "psych yourself up" when encountering temptation to deviate from your behavior change plan.

Describe three steps for preventing behavior relapse.

What is the danger of setting the extinction of an unwanted behavior as a goal?

What is the benefit of having a trial period for a behavior change plan?

Describe the rationale behind avoiding problem situations in the early phases of behavior change.

What is contingency management?

Describe the term behavior chains.

1) Asserting yourself can help in many situations. Learn to say "no, thank you" to people and temptations.
2) In social situations, practice choosing foods according to your plan rather than other people's choices.
3) Practice stopping negative thoughts about yourself; focus on positive ones.

Sensory appeal such as flavor, appearance, and odor are most significant in directing food choices. Secondary factors include health value, expediency, energy value, and cost.

Striving for the extinction of a behavior may not be realistic. Focusing on reducing the frequency of the behavior may make a person less likely to become discouraged.

To prevent relapse:

1) identify high risk situations
2) mentally rehearse a response to potential lapses,
3) remind yourself of the original reasons for making the commitment to change

Avoiding situations that are particularly tempting may be necessary at first until new habits are firmly established.

Contemplating a lifestyle change and the commitment involved may be initially overwhelming. Planning a 6- to 8-week trial period can make a goal seem more attainable and thus increase confidence.

Behavior chains are linked or related behaviors. It is important to control behavior chains that lead to the behavior one wants to change, such as visiting an all-you-can-eat restaurant and then overeating.

Contingency management involves planning in advance for failures so that when disruptive situations arise, one can react constructively.

Is it possible to separate totally the diseases of anorexia nervosa and bulimia nervosa?

Define the term bulimia nervosa.

What is the hallmark of this disease?

What are the two major health problems associated with bulimia nervosa?

Define the term anorexia nervosa.

What is the hallmark of this disease?

Outline the treatment for bulimia nervosa.

Outline the basic treatment for anorexia nervosa.

List three potential health problems caused by anorexia nervosa.

What is the profile of the typical person with bulimia nervosa?

Bulimia nervosa is a disorder in which the person binges on large amounts of food and then tries to purge those calories by fasting, vomiting, exercise, or other means. The hallmark of the disease is the binge-purge cycle.

No, the diseases anorexia nervosa and bulimia nervosa considerably overlap. People with anorexia nervosa might go through stages of bingeing and purging, whereas those with bulimia nervosa might go through stages of semistarvation.

Anorexia nervosa is a psychological disorder in which the person loses significant amounts of weight and ends up essentially "skin and bones." The hallmark of the disease is a refusal to consume enough energy to support energy needs.

1) If the person purges by vomiting, teeth become demineralized and may require extraction.

2) Blood potassium often decreases because vomit contains much potassium. This can cause problems in heart rhythm and even lead to sudden death.

Treatment of anorexia nervosa requires professional help, especially psychological therapy. In the initial stages, refeeding the person is important to regain physical energy and decrease the mental preoccupation with food.

Treatment for bulimia nervosa includes psychotherapy, primarily to help the person acquire a better sense of body image and self-image. The nutritional emphasis is on regular eating habits, not on stopping and bingeing and purging. Once regular eating habits are established, the bingeing and purging cycle should stop by itself.

The individual is usually a college-age woman and probably has been on many weight reduction diets since her teenage years. She is usually only slightly overweight.

Potential health problems include 1) decreased body temperature, 2) decreased heart rate, 3) anemia, 4) low white blood cell count, 5) constipation, 6) low blood potassium, 7) loss of menstruation, 8) bone loss, and 9) possibly heart failure.

Name three causes of death associated with anorexia nervosa.

What are three sources of false messages concerning the "ideal" body?

What are the three different eating patterns seen in binge eating disorder?

What are two main factors that contribute to the onset of anorexia nervosa?

Repeated vomiting can have what three adverse affects on the body?

Describe the female athlete triad.

What are the typical social characteristics of a person with anorexia nervosa?

What are aspects of the psychological profile?

Define the term baryophobia.

What causes this disease?

Sources include the following:

1) TV programs
2) billboard ads
3) magazines
4) movies
5) newspapers

1) suicide

2) heart ailments

3) infections

1) Adolescents' need for acceptance from parents and peers causes them to react intensely to how they think others perceive them.

2) Adolescent body changes are beyond the control of teens and they seek a way to keep control over their bodies.

1) continually eating over a defined period of time, called grazing

2) cycles of bingeing interspersed with normal eating

3) eating normally until an emotional setback occurs, and then eating large amounts of food

Female athlete triad is characterized by the following:

- disordered eating
- low bone density
- lack of menstrual periods

Affects of repeated vomiting include the following:

1) demineralization of teeth

2) lowered blood potassium that can disturb the hearts rhythm

3) swollen, infected salivary glands

4) stomach ulcers

5) tears in the esophagus

Baryophobia--or fear of fat--is a relatively new disorder found in children and is characterized by poor growth. This poor growth usually results from parents underfeeding their children because they fear their children may develop early stages of heart disease or become obese.

The person generally comes from a higher socioeconomic class, may participate in physical activity such as ballet and gymnastics, or work as a model. The person generally sees herself as fat although she is thin and often thinks her stomach protrudes.

What is the difference between an embryo and a fetus?

What is the major difference between the diets for a pregnant woman and a breastfeeding woman?

How does the fetus receive nourishment?

What are two goals of a successful pregnancy that pertain to the infant?

When is the best time for a woman to focus on good nutritional habits to increase chances for having a healthy baby?

What are the two most important factors that influence infant birth weight?

What are three abnormalities seen in infants with fetal alcohol syndrome (FAS)?

Name two conditions that develop more frequently in low-birth-weight infants.

The breastfeeding diet is basically the same as that in pregnancy, with the exception of increased calcium, fluid, and energy needs; an extra glass of milk suffices.

In humans, embryo refers to the offspring developing in utero from about the beginning of the third week to the end of the eighth week after conception.

Two goals for a successful pregnancy regarding the infant are a gestational period longer than 37 weeks and a birth weight greater than 2500 grams (5½ pounds).

The mother nourishes her offspring via the placenta.

Environmental factors such as smoking and nutritional factors such as the mother's weight gain have the most influence on birth weight outcome. Genetics has less of an effect.

Months before a woman becomes pregnant is the ideal time to focus on nutrition. Good nutritional practices are especially critical throughout a woman's childbearing years.

Low-birth-weight infants are at a great risk for infections, other illnesses, physical problems, and death.

Heavy or regular alcohol use during pregnancy can result in poor fetal and later infant growth, physical abnormalities, and mental retardation.

What is the most critical time period with respect to fetal development?

Why is fasting or "crash" dieting dangerous for fetal development?

How many additional kilocalories are needed as a result of pregnancy?

What risk is increased by maternal smoking, alcohol consumption, imprudent medication use, and illegal drug use during pregnancy?

What is potentially harmful about the "eating for two" concept some pregnant women have?

What mineral need of pregnancy can only be met with a supplement?

What is the recommended weight gain during pregnancy?

Using the Food Guide Pyramid, outline a recommended diet during pregnancy.

A pregnant woman will develop ketosis if food intake is greatly restricted. Ketone bodies are thought to be poorly used by the fetal brain and thus restrict brain development.

The first trimester is the most critical period for fetal development. Most organs show great development during this time.

These factors greatly increase the risk of having a premature or small-for-gestational-age infant.

Pregnancy demands an average 300 extra kcal each day in the second and third trimesters.

Iron needs are so high that all women should consider taking a prenatal iron supplement under a physician's guidance.

Although energy and nutrient needs do increase, the mother does not have that many extra kilocalories to use (about 300 per day in the second and third trimesters) for meeting these increased and other nutrient needs.

An adequate diet during pregnancy should include the following servings from each food group:

4 - milk, yogurt, cheese
2 to 3 - meat, poultry, fish, beans
2 to 4 - fruits
3 to 5 - vegetables
6 to 11 - breads, cereals, rice, pasta

The weight gain goal is 25 to 35 pounds for women of healthy body weight. The recommendation is adjusted for underweight and overweight women.

Name the vitamin that might need to be supplemented in the diet of a breastfed infant.

What changes in food habits will ease the problem of constipation in pregnancy?

List two ways a pregnant woman can easily increase her folate intake.

What is the main factor that stimulates human milk production?

Name and describe the first fluid produced by the mother's breast.

Describe the important reflex of the mother that is necessary for breastfeeding.

Why do breastfed infants show typically fewer respiratory and intestinal infections than formula-fed infants?

How can a nursing mother know if her infant is receiving enough milk?

An increased intake of water, dietary fiber, and dried fruits, along with regular physical activity, can help reduce constipation.

Although a form of vitamin D is present in human milk, supplementation is recommended <u>if adequate sunlight exposure cannot be guaranteed</u>.

Infant suckling stimulates the release of the hormone prolactin, which in turn stimulates milk production. The more the infant suckles, the greater is the production of milk.

Choosing folate-rich foods, such as oranges and other raw fruits and vegetables, as well as fortified breakfast cereals, helps meet folate needs. However, many physicians recommend a prenatal supplement to ensure adequate intake.

The "let down" reflex is necessary for the release of milk from storage so it can travel to the nipple.

Colostrum is the type of milk produced for the first few days after birth. It is thick and yellowish and contains immune factors.

One standard is that the breastfed infant should have at least six wet diapers a day and show normal growth.

The antibodies present in colostrum and human milk compensate for the infant's immature immune system.

How should new foods be added to an infant's diet to detect a possible allergy?

At what age do adolescent girls and boys experience a rapid growth spurt?

Name four common allergy-causing foods.

Compare the degree of hunger found in an infant with that found in a preschooler.

What should be the focus when assessing a teenager's snacking habits?

Name two ways parents can help their preschooler develop a healthful eating pattern.

Define the term food intolerance.

Why might a child benefit from being constantly introduced to new foods?

In most girls a growth spurt begins between the ages of 10 and 13 years, whereas in boys it begins between ages 12 and 15 years.

New foods should be introduced singly, not mixed, in 7-day intervals. This allows time to determine if an allergy develops and thus permits the offending food to be easily identified.

Preschoolers normally experience less hunger than they did as infants because of decreased growth rates.

Egg whites, chocolate, nuts, and cow's milk are the most common allergy-causing foods fed to infants.

Parents can set a good example by eating a variety of healthful foods. Encouraging the preschooler to take at least one bite of everything will help ensure variety in the diet.

Snacking is not inherently harmful; the focus should be on what makes up the snack. Wise food choices can make snacks a healthful part of a teenager's diet.

Providing new foods to a child can expand food choices, help develop an experimental approach, and teach the child to enjoy a variety of foods.

A food intolerance is an adverse reaction to food that does not involve an immune process. Most people are less sensitive to their food intolerances than allergic people are to their offending foods.

What historical evidence suggests that nurture is very important for allowing maximal development in childhood?

At what age does a child first attempt self-feeding?

Why would inhibiting cell division, as can result from a poor diet, be so harmful to an infant?

Compare the protein needs of an infant with those of an adult on a per kilogram basis.

Which clinical methods provide useful information on growth and development?

What unit of measurement is used for this method?

Compare the water need of an infant with that of an adult on a per kcal burned basis.

Describe how a food allergy is tested.

How can iron deficiency be prevented in childhood?

About 10 months of age is when an infant practices self-feeding of finger foods and drinking from a cup.

From suits of armor and Egyptian mummies we can tell that adults of the past were smaller than adults today, even though infants were the same size. The poor diets of people in the past did not supply enough nutrients for maximal growth.

Infants need about 2 grams of protein per kilogram of body weight daily. This is more than twice the RDA for adults (0.8 grams per kilogram).

Later improving the diet, once the time for cell division has stopped, will not restore any lack of growth experienced.

Infants need 1.5 milliliters of water per kcal burned or about 150 milliliters per kilogram of body weight. This is 1.5 times more than the needs of an adult (1 milliliter per kcal expended).

The height-for-age and weight-for-height growth charts give useful information in assessing growth and development. Numbers in these charts are expressed in percentiles, which represent the rank of the person among 100 age- and sex-matched peers.

Regular consumption of good iron sources is essential. A few ounces of lean meat and a serving of iron-fortified cereal are generally easy to incorporate into a child's diet.

The first step in detecting a food allergy is to keep a detailed record of symptoms, time from ingestion to onset of symptoms, and suspected foods. Then all suspected foods are removed from the diet and reintroduced singly in small amounts.

What are two causes of failure to thrive?

How often should an infant be burped during breastfeeding or bottle-feeding?

What four factors should be considered when deciding to introduce solid food to an infant's diet?

What is the greatest quantity of formula or milk infants should be fed daily?

At about what age should children be started on solid food?

At what age should bottle-feeding be discontinued?

What is one widespread reason for introducing solid foods earlier than the recommended time?

What is the best age and method to treat childhood obesity?

It is important to burp an infant every 10 minutes while breastfeeding or after 1 to 2 ounces while bottle-feeding.

Physical causes of failure to thrive include chronic diarrhea, infection, and heart problems. However, about half the cases show no disease process and thus may result from poor child-rearing practices, such as inattention to the infant's needs.

Infants should not be fed more than 40 total ounces of formula or 32 total ounces of milk per day. After 6 to 8 months, solid foods in the diet should be increased instead.

One must consider 1) the infant's nutritional needs; 2) physiological readiness, such as kidney function and starch digestion; 3) physical readiness, such as sitting up and head control; and 4) susceptibility to food allergies.

Bottle-feeding should be stopped by 18 months of age.

The American Academy of Pediatrics recommends that solid food not be given to infants until 4 to 6 months of age.

The best time to address obesity is in childhood because adolescent obesity most likely leads to adult obesity. The first step is to assess the child's activity pattern. Moderation in energy intake is important; weight-loss diets are usually not necessary for young children.

Many people believe early introduction of solid food will help an infant sleep through the night. However, this ability is a developmental milestone and has little relation to what an infant eats before going to bed.

Describe the autoimmune theory of cellular aging.

Why should many nutritional recommendations for health be individualized?

Name two significant drug-nutrient interactions that often exist in the elderly.

What have animal experiments with low-energy diets revealed about the link between aging and diet?

Describe our current understanding of nutrient needs of the elderly.

Why is it important to make sure elderly people consume enough water?

Name three nutrients that deserve special emphasis in a diet plan for the elderly.

What is the main intestinal problem found in the elderly? How should it be treated with diet?

Since the response to different components is often idiosyncratic, dietary recommendations, such as for sodium, should be made on an individual basis to be most valid.

Autoimmune reactions occur when antibodies and white blood cells cannot distinguish between foreign compounds and your own body. Thus your immune system attacks your body tissue as well as foreign compounds. This can kill cells and in turn lead to some effects of aging.

In experiments, animals that were raised on two-thirds the energy they would normally consume lived 35% longer than those freely fed. This suggests that a slowing of the aging process may be linked to a restricted energy intake.

Drug-related nutritional problems include an increased need for potassium when using some types of diuretics and changes in appetite when certain antibiotics are used.

Partial loss of the sense of thirst typically occurs among the elderly. This puts them at a greater risk for dehydration, which can lead to confusion.

Scientists have only recently started to study this area extensively. Most recommendations are made using extrapolations from adult needs.

Many elderly persons suffer from constipation. They should gradually increase their dietary fiber intake to about 35 grams daily. Fluid intake should also increase to prevent intestinal blockage from the high fiber intake.

The elderly need to emphasize adequate intakes of vitamin D (or sun exposure), vitamin B-6, vitamin B-12, calcium, and zinc.

What are the two principal causes of death in Western society today?

Name two examples of community nutrition programs for the elderly.

What two basic processes cause the aging of cells?

How is the immune system affected by aging and diet?

What two nutrients are needed for immune function?

Describe how both errors in DNA replication and damage by free radicals can cause cells to age.

How does lifestyle affect muscle mass throughout adult years?

What are four symptoms of Alzheimer's disease?

Nutritional problems in a person with alcoholism result from deficiencies of a variety of nutrients. Name four nutrients commonly deficient in persons with alcoholism.

Nutrition programs for the elderly include congregate meals where elderly people gather for lunch, home delivery of meals, food cooperatives, and programs of many social organizations.

Heart disease and cancer are linked with most deaths in contemporary Western society.

The immune system becomes less efficient with age; adequate <u>protein</u> and <u>zinc</u> intakes are needed to maximize its function. Consuming animal proteins is one way to obtain these nutrients.

Aging of cells is probably a result of both <u>automatic</u> cellular changes and <u>environmental</u> influences.

Lifestyle partly determines the rate of muscle mass deterioration. An active lifestyle helps maintain muscle mass, whereas an inactive lifestyle causes a loss of muscle mass.

1) Enough errors are made in DNA replication to prevent the cell from producing the proteins necessary for functioning, and therefore the cell dies.

2) Free radicals can attack cell membranes and proteins, in turn leading to cell death.

Choose: vitamin A,
thiamin,
niacin,
vitamin B-6,
folate,
vitamin D,
vitamin C,
vitamin K

1) Personality change

2) Unreasonable fears

3) Outbursts

4) General forgetfulness

According to recent research, how do the RDAs compare with the best estimates of the needs of the elderly?

Define life expectancy.

What is the life expectancy for men and women in the United States?

Heart attack and stroke--the major causes of death in all adults--are caused primarily by atherosclerosis and high blood pressure. Define atherosclerosis and tell how it can be controlled.

What is osteoporosis and why is this commonly seen in elderly?

Describe a plan for prevention.

How can depression and mental state affect nutritional status?

List three practical suggestions for diet planning for single elderly people.

List four reasons good nutrition is such a benefit to the elderly.

What are the recommendations for alcohol intake established by most health organizations?

Life expectancy is the time an average person born in a specific year can expect to live. Life expectancy in America is 73 years for men and about 80 years for women.

For healthy elderly people, the RDA is probably too high for vitamin A; too low for protein (active elders), vitamin D, B-6, B-12, and calcium; and about right for the other nutrients.

Osteoporosis is the decline in bone density associated with aging. It most commonly occurs in women, especially after menopause. At least meeting the RDA for calcium can help build and maintain density in some types of bones. However, estrogen therapy at menopause for women is the best way to prevent bone loss in the spine.

Atherosclerosis is the process of accumulating plaque in the arteries, reducing their elasticity, constricting blood flow, and consequently elevating blood pressure. Use diet (and possibly medications) to keep blood cholesterol below 200 mg/dl and blood pressure within normal limits. Also, don't smoke.

1) If you have a freezer, cook large amounts, divide into portions, and freeze.

2) Ask the grocer to break open a family-sized package of wrapped meat or vegetables.

3) Buy only several pieces of fruit - perhaps a ripe one, a medium-ripe one, and a green one - so that they will ripen over a period of several days.

Depression can lead to a downward spiral in which poor appetite produces weakness that leads to even poorer appetite. The resulting poor nutritional state can produce further mental confusion, increased isolation, and loneliness.

Experts generally recommend limiting alcohol consumption to the equivalent of less than 1 ounce of pure alcohol in a single day. This is equivalent to two cans of beer, two small glasses of wine, or two average cocktails.

1) Delays some disease progression
2) Improves management of existing diseases
3) Increases mental, physical, and social well being
4) Decreases the need for and length of hospitalization

CHAPTER 17

How does the amount of an additive allowed in a food compare with the amount found safe in animal studies?

Name three naturally occurring toxins in food.

What does the Delaney Clause state?

How can variety and moderation in food selection protect against both naturally occurring and environmental food toxins?

Name two functions of antioxidants in foods.

What are three common antioxidants?

What responsibilities concerning food fall under the jurisdiction of the Food and Drug Administration (FDA)?

What are sulfites, and why must they be specially regulated by the FDA?

How does irradiation act to preserve food?

Some potentially harmful chemicals that occur naturally include aflatoxin, goitrogens, tannins, oxalic acid, solanine, and nitrates.

After scientists determine the highest dose of an additive that produces no ill effects in test animals, that amount is then divided by at least 100 to establish the amount allowed to be added to human food.

Variety and moderation in food selection help ensure that you are not consuming too much of any one food that may contain a contaminant. The frequency of exposure to any potentially toxin-laden food is thus decreased.

The Delaney Clause prohibits the intentional addition of cancer-causing compounds in foods under FDA jurisdiction.

The Food and Drug Administration (FDA) ensures the safety and wholesomeness of all foods sold through interstate commerce, except for meat and poultry, which are under USDA jurisdiction. FDA sets standards and then enforces the regulations.

Antioxidants help delay discoloration of foods and help prevent fats from becoming rancid. BHA, BHT, and vitamins E and C are widely used antioxidants.

Food irradiation creates free radicals in food, which can destroy cell membranes and attack DNA and proteins. By doing so, irradiation can prevent the growth of microorganisms, parasites, and insects.

Sulfites and sulfur-containing compounds prevent food discoloration. However, since some people are sensitive to sulfites and react with wheezing, hives, diarrhea, and other symptoms, FDA has prohibited their use on raw fruits and vegetables, except potatoes.

Describe how Salmonella bacteria usually enter foods.

Can refrigeration stop the growth of all bacteria?

In what temperature range should cooked foods be stored?

Name three methods of food preservation that have been used for centuries.

What treatment is recommended for diarrhea associated with food-borne illness?

What are the two basic ways in which food spoils?

Name three types of preservatives.

Describe the action of emulsifiers in foods.

No, some bacteria can grow even at refrigeration temperatures.

Salmonella bacteria are found in human and animal feces and enter the food chain via infected water, contaminated cutting boards, cracked eggs, and pieces of feces in food.

Past methods of food preservation include use of smoke, salt, sugar, fermentation, and drying.

Store cooked foods below 40° F (4° C) or above 140° F (60° C). This helps avoid holding foods in the moderate temperature range in which microbes flourish.

Food spoilage can occur from the following:

1) bacterial, viral, or fungal contamination

2) exposure to oxygen

The person should drink plenty of fluids. To prevent further contamination, hands should be washed frequently and food handling should be temporarily avoided or at least minimized.

Emulsifiers suspend fat in water, preventing their separation. This often improves uniformity, texture, and body of a food.

Preservatives may be in the form of the following:

1) antioxidants
2) inhibitors of microbial growth
3) sequestrants which bind free metal ions

In what environment does Clostridium botulinum thrive?

Contrast intentional and incidental food additives.

Why are signs of spoilage on commercially canned foods, such as rust on seams, holes, and swollen sides, so dangerous?

What precautions should be taken if such spoilage is seen?

What is the GRAS list?

Why was it established?

Define the term pasteurization.

What causes the greatest health risk from the food we eat: microbes or additives?

What two mechanisms do bacteria use to cause food-borne illness?

Describe how Staphylococcus aureus usually enters foods.

Intentional additives are directly and purposefully put into food. Incidental additives are those that may reasonably be expected to become components of food during processing or packaging. Both are regulated by FDA.

Clostridium botulinum are anaerobic bacteria and thus can only grow in absence of air. Improperly home canned food and foods with an anaerobic center, such as potato salad, can become contaminated.

The generally recognized as safe (GRAS) list was established in 1958 by the U.S. Congress. All food additives in use in the United States that were considered safe were put on the list so that manufacturers would not needlessly have to prove their safety.

Signs of spoilage in commercially canned foods may indicate contamination by the anaerobic bacteria Clostridium botulinum. Do not taste the food. If Clostridium botulinum is present, the toxins could cause a fatal result. Simply discard the product.

Contamination by bacteria and to a lesser extent by molds, fungi, and viruses poses the greatest health risk from food.

Pasteurization is a partial sterilization process that uses high temperatures for a short time to destroy microbes.

Staphylococcus aureus bacteria live in nasal passages and the skin. When people sneeze or cough over food or people with open sores handle food, the bacteria can enter the food.

Bacteria can do either of the following:

1) directly invade the intestine, in turn introducing toxins that are part of the cells themselves

2) produce toxins to cause food-borne illness

Describe three critical periods in human development.

Define the term malnutrition.

Define the term undernutrition.

This is mainly linked to what social factor?

Define the term protein-energy malnutrition.

Name five symptoms of chronic undernutrition.

What does the World Health Organization (WHO) mean by the term "silent undernutrition"?

List four factors that currently contribute to undernutrition in the developing world.

Describe the School Breakfast and Lunch programs.

Malnutrition is a condition of impaired development or function caused by a long-term deficiency, excess, or imbalance of energy intake and/or nutrients.

Critical periods are times when the human organism is particularly susceptible to the effects of undernutrition because of rapid growth. These include pregnancy, infancy, and childhood.

Protein-energy malnutrition is a form of undernutrition caused by an extremely deficient intake of energy, protein, or both.

Undernutrition is the malnutrition that results from an inadequate intake, absorption, or utilization of the nutrients or energy needed for optimal growth, development, and body function.

Poverty is its major cause.

The term silent undernutrition is reflected in the young child whose weight is several pounds below the low end of the normal range on a growth chart. The untrained eye may miss this condition or simply see the child as being skinny.

1. tiredness
2. muscle soreness
3. irritability
4. edema
5. hunger pains

Both the School Lunch and Breakfast Programs enable low-income schoolchildren to receive meals at reduced cost or no cost if certain income guidelines are met.

1. inadequate food supplies
2. war/civil unrest
3. depletion of natural resources
4. poor infrastructure for food production and health maintenance
5. external debt
6. cultural attitudes towards certain foods

Describe the special supplemental feeding program for Women, Infants, and Children (WIC).

What did Thomas Malthus predict about the eventual course of the food/population ratio?

Outline a key step to ending hunger worldwide.

Define the term green revolution.

Name four benefits of using human milk for infant feeding in countries of the developing world.

Name three reasons for poor sanitation conditions in countries of the developing world.

Define the term biotechnology.

List a key policy to reduce famine worldwide.

Malthus predicted the population would increase faster than the food supply and so the population will eventually outgrow the food supply.

The WIC program provides food vouchers and nutrition education to low-income pregnant and lactating women and their young children.

The term green revolution describes a phenomenon starting in the 1960s where a dramatic rise in crop yields in some countries, such as the Philippines, India, and Mexico, was made possible because of increased use of fertilizers and development of superior crops through careful plant breeding.

Providing employment opportunities for all who desire to work is a key step to ending hunger worldwide.

1. human feces
2. rotting garbage
3. insect and rodent infestations

Human milk is hygienic, readily available, and nutritionally sound and provides immune factors.

Policies to prevent famine focus on reducing war and civil strife. Increasing the productivity of rural people is also important.

Biotechnology, also known as genetic engineering, used a wide range of cells and subcell technology for synthesizing and then placing genetic material in organisms.